MEDICAL MARIJUANA
AND MARIJUANA USE

MEDICAL MARIJUANA AND MARIJUANA USE

ALBERT T. JOHNSON
EDITOR

Nova Science Publishers, Inc.
New York

Copyright © 2009 by Nova Science Publishers, Inc.

LIBRARY OF CONGRESS CATALOGING-IN-PUBLICATION DATA
Available upon request
ISBN: 978-1-60692-899-8

Published by Nova Science Publishers, Inc. ✤ *New York*

CONTENTS

PREFACE

Twelve states, mostly in the West, have enacted laws allowing the use of marijuana for medical purposes, and many thousands of patients are seeking relief from a variety of serious illnesses by smoking marijuana or using other herbal cannabis preparations. Meanwhile, the federal Drug Enforcement Administration refuses to recognize these state laws and continues to investigate and arrest, under federal statute, medical marijuana providers and users in those states and elsewhere. Claims and counterclaims about medical marijuana — much debated by journalists and academics, policymakers at all levels of government, and interested citizens — include the following: Marijuana is harmful and has no medical value; marijuana effectively treats the symptoms of certain diseases; smoking is an improper route of drug administration; marijuana should be rescheduled to permit medical use; state medical marijuana laws send the wrong message and lead to increased illicit drug use; the medical marijuana movement undermines the war on drugs; patients should not be arrested for using medical marijuana; the federal government should allow the states to experiment and should not interfere with state medical marijuana programs; medical marijuana laws harm the federal drug approval process; the medical cannabis movement is a cynical ploy to legalize marijuana and other drugs. With strong opinions being expressed on all sides of this complex issue, the debate over medical marijuana does not appear to be approaching resolution.

Chapter 1 - This Chartbook recognizes marijuana as a major component of the illicit drug problem. Major progress has been achieved in reducing youth marijuana use; nevertheless, the overall demand for marijuana remains strong.

The supply of cannabis is complex, involving domestic and foreign growers — both outdoor and indoor — as well as intricate networks that involve not only conventional drug traffickers, but also established social networks of friends and family. The potency of cannabis has risen dramatically in the past two decades, with concomitant abuse and dependence consequences reflected in increasing cannabis-related emergency and treatment events.

Chapter 2 - The issue before Congress is whether to continue the federal prosecution of medical marijuana patients and their providers, in accordance with the federal Controlled Substances Act (CSA), or whether to relax federal marijuana prohibition enough to permit the medicinal use of botanical cannabis products when recommended by a physician, especially where permitted under state law.

The first action on medical marijuana in the current Congress occurred in April 2007, at markup of the Prescription Drug User Fee Act (S. 1082). The Senate Committee on Health, Education, Labor, and Pensions adopted an amendment, not included in the enacted bill, requiring "that State-legalized medical marijuana be subject to the full regulatory requirements of the Food and Drug Administration." Then, in July 2007, the Hinchey-Rohrabacher amendment to prevent federal enforcement of the CSA against medical marijuana users and providers in the states that have legalized its use was rejected by the full House by a vote of 165 to 262.

In: Medical Marijuana and Marijuana Use   ISBN 978-1-60692-899-8
Editor: Albert T. Johnson   © 2009 Nova Science Publishers, Inc.

Chapter 1

2008 MARIJUANA SOURCEBOOK: MARIJUANA: THE GREATEST CAUSE OF ILLEGAL DRUG ABUSE[*]

Office of National Drug Control Policy

INTRODUCTION

This article recognizes marijuana as a major component of the illicit drug problem. Major progress has been achieved in reducing youth marijuana use; nevertheless, the overall demand for marijuana remains strong.

The supply of cannabis is complex, involving domestic and foreign growers — both outdoor and indoor — as well as intricate networks that involve not only conventional drug traffickers, but also established social networks of friends and family. The potency of cannabis has risen dramatically in the past two decades, with concomitant abuse and dependence consequences reflected in increasing cannabis-related emergency and treatment events.

Today, in addition to traditional methods of promoting and consuming the drug, marijuana is being marketed as candy to young people, the next generation of potential buyers.

---

[*] This is an edited, excerpted and augmented edition of a Office of National Drug Control Policy, Washington, DC publication.

The data summary on these pages looks at marijuana use patterns and trends, health effects, criminal justice aspects, the supply network, and the issue of so-called medical marijuana.

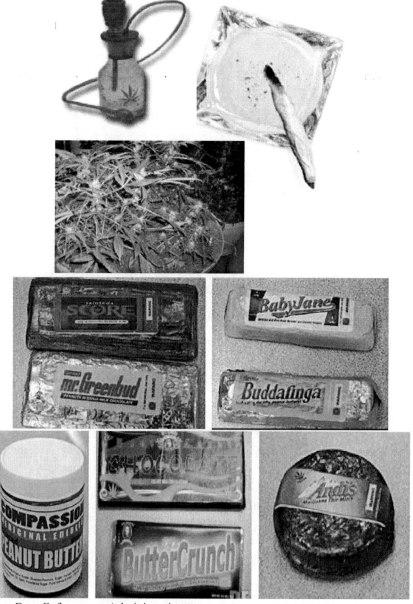

Photos: Drug Enforcement Administration.

USE PATTERNS AND TRENDS

14.8 million Americans were current (past month) users of marijuana in 2006.

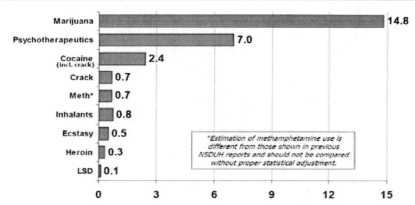

Source: SAMHSA, 2006 National Survey on Drug Use and Health (September 2007).

Figure 1. Marijuana Is the Most Commonly Used Illicit Drug.

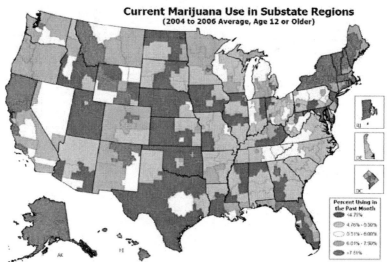

Source: SAMHSA, Substate Estimates from the 2004-2006 National Surveys on Drug Use and Health (June 2008).

Figure 2. Marijuana Use Rates Vary Across the Country.

Marijuana use rates accelerate to a peak at age 20, with one in five reporting current use of marijuana.

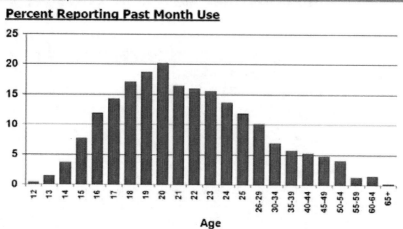

Source: SAMHSA, 2006 National Survey on Drug Use and Health (September 2007).

Figure 3. Age Variability in Marijuana Use.

Trends in Current Use of Marijuana

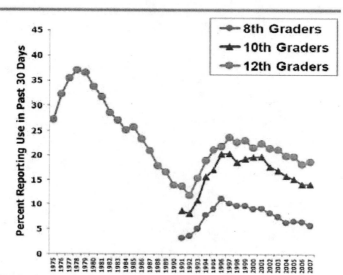

Source: 2007 Monitoring the Future (MTF) study, December 2007.

Figure 4. Marijuana Use Among Youth.

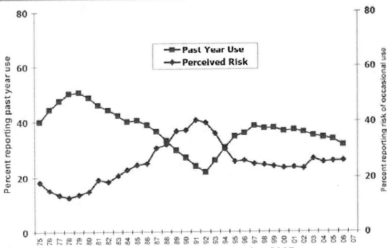

Source: 2007 Monitoring the Future study (MTF), December 2007.

Figure 5. Higher Rates of Perceived Harmfulness of Marijuana Are Associated with Lower Rates of Use.

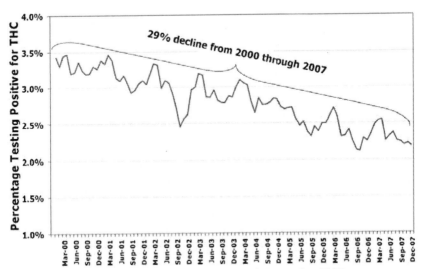

Source: Quest Diagnostics Drug Testing Index, Through December 2007.

Figure 6. Percentage of National Workforce Testing Positive for Marijuana Is Declining.

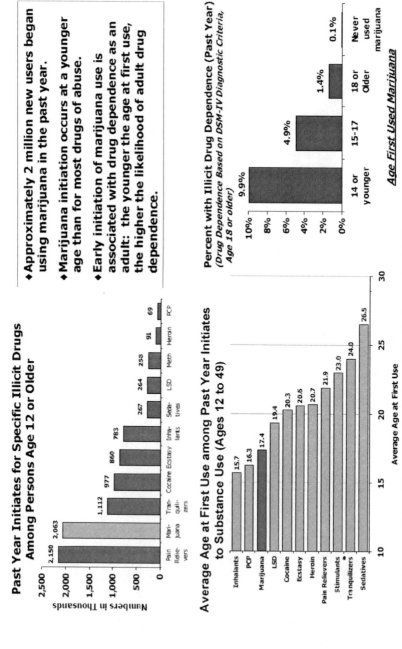

Past Year Initiates for Specific Illicit Drugs Among Persons Age 12 or Older

◆ Approximately 2 million new users began using marijuana in the past year.

◆ Marijuana initiation occurs at a younger age than for most drugs of abuse.

◆ Early initiation of marijuana use is associated with drug dependence as an adult: the younger the age at first use, the higher the likelihood of adult drug dependence.

Percent with Illicit Drug Dependence (Past Year)
(Drug Dependence Based on DSM-IV Diagnostic Criteria, Age 18 or older)

Age First Used Marijuana

Average Age at First Use among Past Year Initiates to Substance Use (Ages 12 to 49)

Source: SAMHSA, 2006 National Survey on Drug Use and Health (September 2007).

Figure 7. Initiation of Marijuana Use.

HEALTH EFFECTS

More Than 4 Million Persons Estimated to be Dependent or Abusers of Marijuana in the Past Year

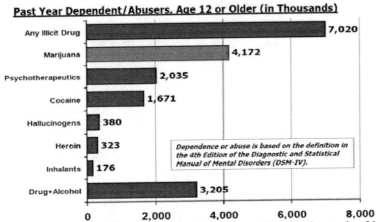

Source: SAMHSA, 2006 National Survey on Drug Use and Health (September 2007).

Figure 8. A Major Consequence Marijuana Use Is the Risk of Dependence or Abuse.

Steady Increase in Treatment Admissions with Marijuana as the Primary Substance of Abuse Since 1994

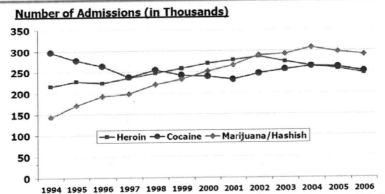

Source: SAMHSA, Treatment Episode Data Set (TEDS) Highlights – 2006 (January 2008); data for 1994 and 1995 are from the 2004 and 2005 TEDS reports, respectively.

Figure 9. Growing Need for Marijuana Treatment.

Treatment Admissions with Marijuana as the Primary Substance of Abuse

All Admissions

Ages 12 to 17

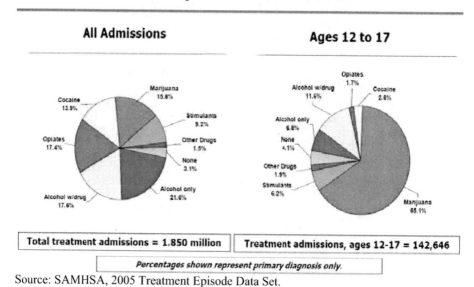

| Total treatment admissions = 1.850 million | Treatment admissions, ages 12-17 = 142,646 |

Percentages shown represent primary diagnosis only.

Source: SAMHSA, 2005 Treatment Episode Data Set.

Figure 10. Youth Are in Treatment Primarily for Marijuana.

Use and Dependence/Abuse for Ages 12 to 17

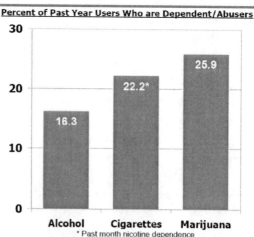

Percent of Past Year Users Who are Dependent/Abusers

* Past month nicotine dependence

Source: SAMHSA, 2006 National Survey on Drug Use and Health (September 2007).

Figure 11. For Younger Users, Marijuana Is More Addictive and More Dangerous.

According to NSDUH, one in four 12– to 17-year-olds who report using marijuana in the past year display the characteristics of abuse or dependency. For younger users, the risk of marijuana abuse or dependency exceeds that for alcohol or tobacco. Recent research supports the "gateway" dimension of marijuana — that its use creates greater risk of abuse or dependency on other drugs, such as heroin and cocaine. Marijuana use itself is a serious risk, not only for addiction, but also is an added risk for developing psychosis, including schizophrenia.

Emergency department episodes involving marijuana almost tripled from 1994 to 2002. Marijuana steadily increased over that decade, surpassing heroin — which remained relatively flat — in 1998.

Marijuana use is associated with depression, suicidal thoughts, and suicide attempts. Besides the links to depression shown below, teens who smoke marijuana at least once a month are three times more likely to have suicidal thoughts than non-users.

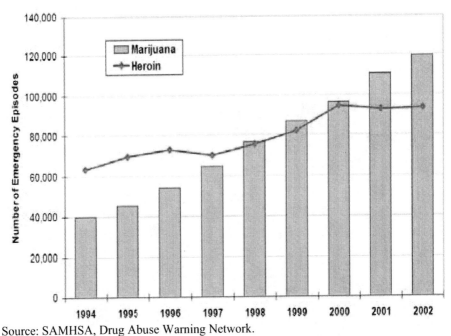

Source: SAMHSA, Drug Abuse Warning Network.

Figure 12. The Burden on Emergency Departments Has Been Increasing.

Ages 12 to 17, Past Year

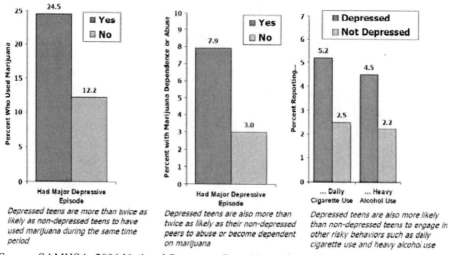

Depressed teens are more than twice as likely as non-depressed teens to have used marijuana during the same time period

Depressed teens are also more than twice as likely as their non-depressed peers to abuse or become dependent on marijuana

Depressed teens are also more likely than non-depressed teens to engage in other risky behaviors such as daily cigarette use and heavy alcohol use

Source: SAMHSA, 2006 National Survey on Drug Use and Health (September 2007).

Figure 13. Marijuana Use Is Associated with Mental Health Disorders.

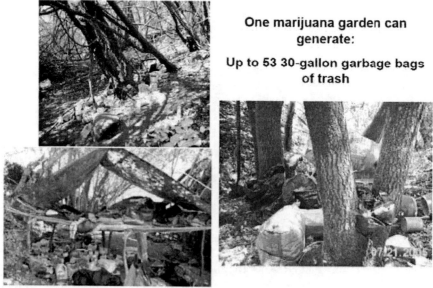

One marijuana garden can generate:

Up to 53 30-gallon garbage bags of trash

Photos: Campaign Against Marijuana Planting (2005).

Figure 14. Marijuana Growers Present Environmental Hazards.

CRIMINAL JUSTICE ASPECTS

Youth who engage in anti-social behavior are far more likely to use marijuana than those who do not engage in these behaviors.

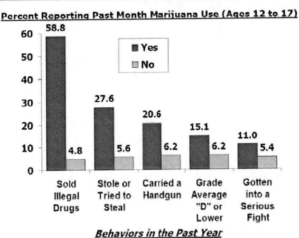

Source: SAMHSA, 2006 National Survey on Drug Use and Health (September 2007).

Figure 15. Juvenile Delinquent Behavior Is Closely Associated With Marijuana Use.

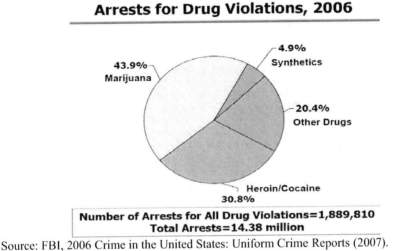

Source: FBI, 2006 Crime in the United States: Uniform Crime Reports (2007).

Figure 16. Marijuana Accounts for Two Out of Five Arrests for Drug Violations.

Inmates in State Prisons

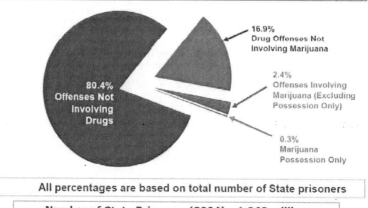

16.9%
Drug Offenses Not
Involving Marijuana

2.4%
Offenses Involving
Marijuana (Excluding
Possession Only)

0.3%
Marijuana
Possession Only

80.4%
Offenses Not
Involving
Drugs

All percentages are based on total number of State prisoners

Number of State Prisoners (2004) =1.262 million

Source: Bureau of Justice Statistics, Prisoners in 2004 (October 2005) and 2004 Survey of
Inmates in State Correctional Facilities, Unpublished tabulations (February 2008).

Figure 17. However, Marijuana Arrests Do Not Translate to a Large Share of Offenders in
Prison.

Source of Referral to Treatment

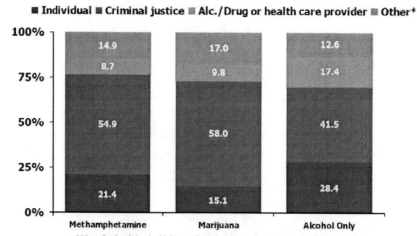

■ Individual ■ Criminal justice ■ Alc./Drug or health care provider ■ Other*

*Other referrals include school (educational), employer/EAP, and other community referrals.

Source: SAMHSA, 2006 Treatment Episode Data Set.

Figure 18. Substantial Proportions of Treatment Referrals for Marijuana,
Methamphetamine, and Alcohol Are from the Criminal Justice System.

Marijuana Users Spent an Estimated $11 Billion to Obtain Marijuana

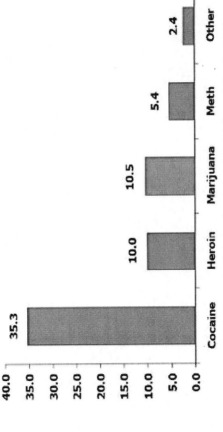

U.S. Users Spent a Total of $64 Billion on Illegal Drugs in 2000

Billions of Dollars (Projection)

Cocaine	Heroin	Marijuana	Meth	Other
35.3	10.0	10.5	5.4	2.4

Source: ONDCP, *What America's Users Spend on Illegal Drugs* (December 2001).

Source:ONDCP, What America's Users Spend on Illegal Drugs (December 20001).

Figure 19. What Marijuana Users Spend.

Method of Obtaining Most Recently Used Marijuana Among Past Year Users

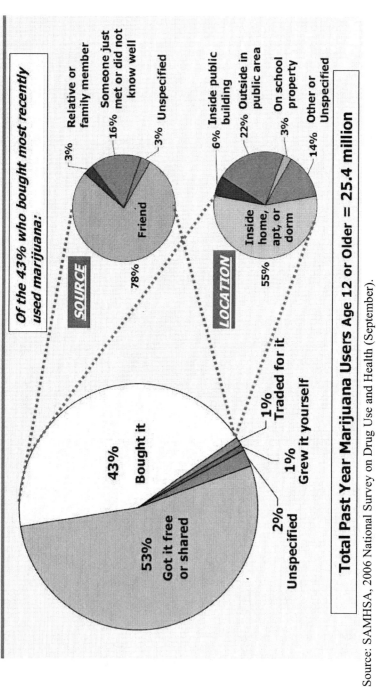

Of the 43% who bought most recently used marijuana:

SOURCE

- 3% Relative or family member
- 16% Someone just met or did not know well
- 3% Unspecified
- 78% Friend

LOCATION

- 6% Inside public building
- 22% Outside in public area
- 3% On school property
- 14% Other or Unspecified
- 55% Inside home, apt, or dorm

- 43% Bought it
- 1% Traded for it
- 1% Grew it yourself
- 2% Unspecified
- 53% Got it free or shared

Total Past Year Marijuana Users Age 12 or Older = 25.4 million

Source: SAMHSA, 2006 National Survey on Drug Use and Health (September).

Figure 20. User Social Networks Are Essential Conduits for Obtaining Marijuana for Individual Use.

Potency of Marijuana Seizures

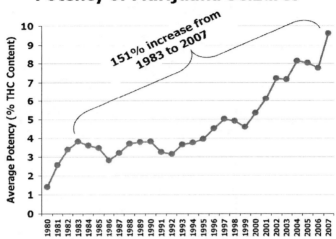

Source: University of Mississippi, National Center for Natural Products Research. Potency Monitoring Project Quarterly Report 100 (April 2008).

Figure 21. Marijuana Potency Has Been Increasing.

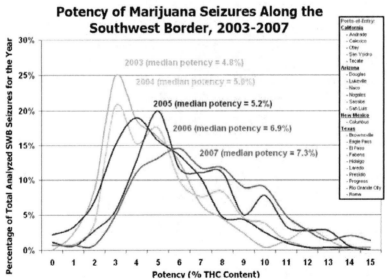

Source: ONDCP analysis of data from the University of Mississippi, Potency Monitoring Project and the Drug Enforcement Administration, System to Retrieve Infromation on Drug Evidence (February 2008).

Figure 22. Marijuana Seizures Along the Southwest Border Are Increasingly More Potent.

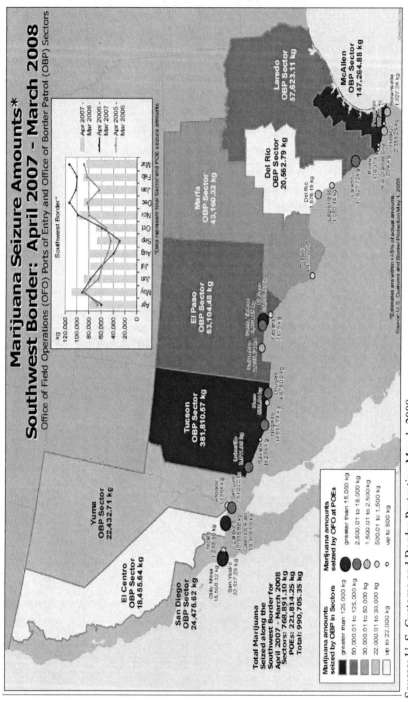

Source: U. S. Customs and Border Protection May 1, 2008.

Figure 23. The Southwest Border is a Key Conduit of Marijuana Supply.

- The largest number of eradicated marijuana plants are concentrated in the West and in Appalachian states
- Although indoor-grown marijuana plants comprise less than 10 percent of total eradicated plants, the quantity is rapidly increasing

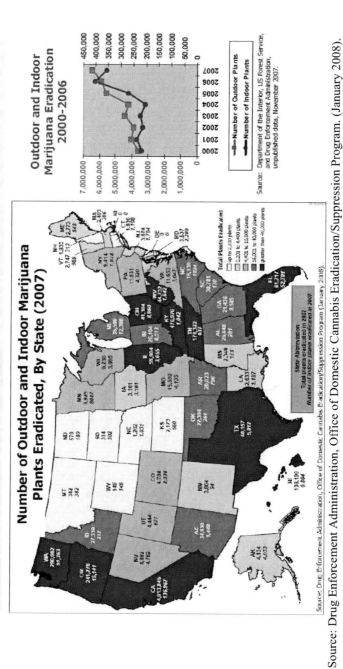

Figure 24. Domestically Grown Marijuana Is a Major Source of Supply.

Source: Drug Enforcement Administration, Office of Domestic Cannabis Eradication/Suppression Program. (January 2008).

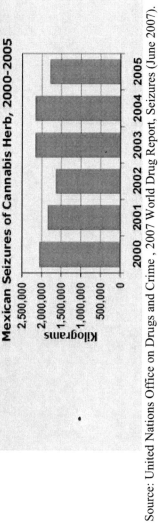

Source: United Nations Office on Drugs and Crime , 2007 World Drug Report, Seizures (June 2007).

Figure 25. Mexico Is a Major Marijuana Producer.

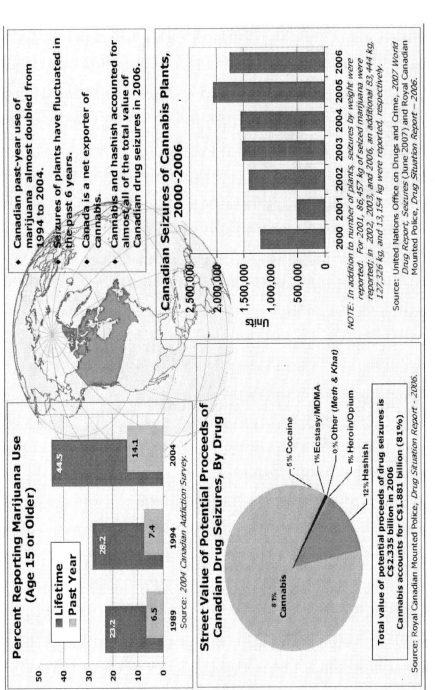

Figure 26. Canada Is a Consumer as Well as a Producer of Marijuana.

The 'Medical Marijuana' Issue

Smoked Marijuana Is Not Medicine

In April 2006, the Food and Drug Administration (FDA) issued an interagency advisory stating that it has not approved smoked marijuana for any medical condition or disease indication. FDA's drug approval process requires well-controlled clinical trials that provide the necessary scientific data upon which FDA makes its approval and labeling decisions, consistent with the standards of the Federal Food, Drug, and Cosmetic Act. New drugs must be shown to be safe and effective for their intended use before being marketed in this country. Efforts that seek to bypass the FDA drug approval process might expose patients to unsafe and ineffective drug products. A growing number of states have passed voter referenda or legislative initiatives making smoked marijuana available for a variety of medical conditions upon a doctor's recommendation. These measures are deemed by FDA to be inconsistent with efforts to ensure that medications undergo the rigorous scientific scrutiny of the approval process. Accordingly, FDA, along with the Drug Enforcement Administration and the Office of National Drug Control Policy, do not support the use of smoked marijuana for medical purposes.

What Did the Institute of Medicine Conclude?

The Institute of Medicine (IOM) reviewed the scientific evidence for the potential benefits and risks associated with marijuana and makes a clear distinction between smoked marijuana and cannabinoids:

- Smoked marijuana is a crude THC delivery system that also delivers harmful substances – hence, smoked marijuana should generally not be recommended for medical use.
- There is potential therapeutic value of cannabinoid drugs for pain relief, control of nausea and vomiting, and appetite stimulation, and this value would be enhanced by a rapid onset of drug effect.
- The future for marijuana as medicine lies in its isolated components – the cannabinoids and their synthetic derivatives. Isolated cannabinoids will provide more reliable effects than crude plant mixtures.

IOM recommends research and clinical trials of cannabinoid drugs and studies of health risks of smoking marijuana.

Source: Institute of Medicine, Marijuana and Medicine: Assessing the Science Base (1999).

Figure 27.

Marijuana Dispensary
Vending Machine
(California 2008)

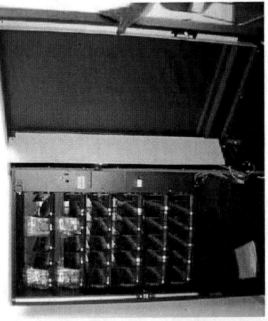

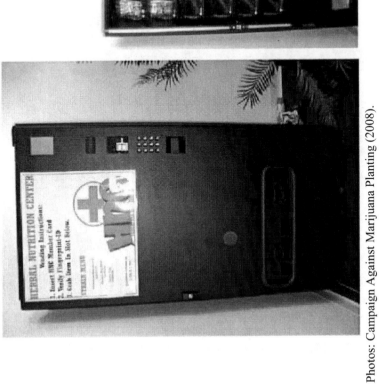

Photos: Campaign Against Marijuana Planting (2008).

Figure 28. Compassionate Care for the Sick and Dying Or Another Front for Drug Trafficking?

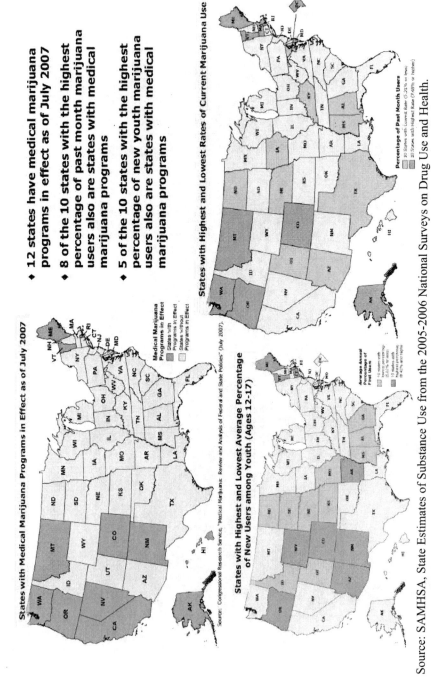

- ◆ 12 states have medical marijuana programs in effect as of July 2007

- ◆ 8 of the 10 states with the highest percentage of past month marijuana users also are states with medical marijuana programs

- ◆ 5 of the 10 states with the highest percentage of new youth marijuana users also are states with medical marijuana programs

Source: SAMHSA, State Estimates of Substance Use from the 2005-2006 National Surveys on Drug Use and Health.

Figure 29. Medical Marijuana States Are More Likely to Have Higher Marijuana Use and Initiation Rates.

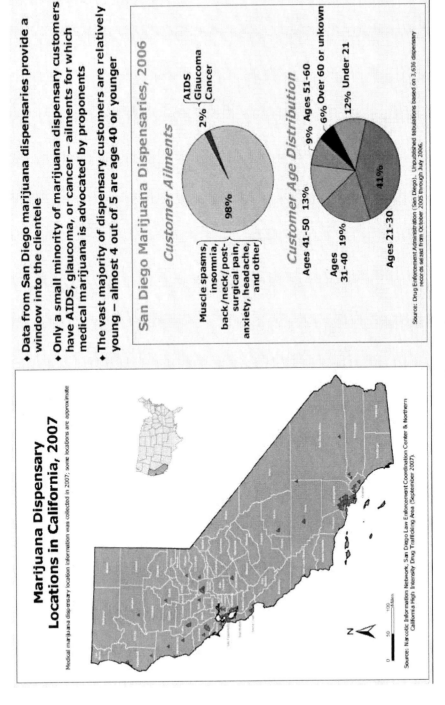

Figure 30. Medical Marijuana Dispensaries in California: A Closer Look.

In: Medical Marijuana and Marijuana Use
Editor: Albert T. Johnson

ISBN 978-1-60692-899-8
© 2009 Nova Science Publishers, Inc.

Chapter 2

MEDICAL MARIJUANA: REVIEW AND ANALYSIS OF FEDERAL AND STATE POLICIES[*]

Mark Eddy

ABSTRACT

The issue before Congress is whether to continue the federal prosecution of medical marijuana patients and their providers, in accordance with the federal Controlled Substances Act (CSA), or whether to relax federal marijuana prohibition enough to permit the medicinal use of botanical cannabis products when recommended by a physician, especially where permitted under state law.

The first action on medical marijuana in the current Congress occurred in April 2007, at markup of the Prescription Drug User Fee Act (S. 1082). The Senate Committee on Health, Education, Labor, and Pensions adopted an amendment, not included in the enacted bill, requiring "that State-legalized medical marijuana be subject to the full regulatory requirements of the Food and Drug Administration." Then, in July 2007, the Hinchey-Rohrabacher amendment to prevent federal enforcement of the CSA against medical marijuana users and providers in the states that have legalized its use was rejected by the full House by a vote of 165 to 262.

In the second session of the current Congress, Representative Barney Frank introduced H.R. 5842, a bill that would allow the medical use of marijuana in states that permit its use with a doctor's recommendation. The

---

[*] This is an edited, excerpted and augmented edition of a CRS Report RL33211, dated June 23, 2008 publication.

Medical Marijuana Patient Protection Act would move marijuana from Schedule I to Schedule II of the CSA and exempt from federal prosecution authorized patients and medical marijuana providers that are acting in accordance with state laws.

Twelve states, mostly in the West, have enacted laws allowing the use of marijuana for medical purposes, and many thousands of patients are seeking relief from a variety of serious illnesses by smoking marijuana or using other herbal cannabis preparations. Meanwhile, the federal Drug Enforcement Administration refuses to recognize these state laws and continues to investigate and arrest, under federal statute, medical marijuana providers and users in those states and elsewhere.

Claims and counterclaims about medical marijuana — much debated by journalists and academics, policymakers at all levels of government, and interested citizens — include the following: Marijuana is harmful and has no medical value; marijuana effectively treats the symptoms of certain diseases; smoking is an improper route of drug administration; marijuana should be rescheduled to permit medical use; state medical marijuana laws send the wrong message and lead to increased illicit drug use; the medical marijuana movement undermines the war on drugs; patients should not be arrested for using medical marijuana; the federal government should allow the states to experiment and should not interfere with state medical marijuana programs; medical marijuana laws harm the federal drug approval process; the medical cannabis movement is a cynical ploy to legalize marijuana and other drugs. With strong opinions being expressed on all sides of this complex issue, the debate over medical marijuana does not appear to be approaching resolution.

INTRODUCTION: THE ISSUE BEFORE CONGRESS

The issue before Congress is whether to continue the federal prosecution of medical marijuana [1] patients and their providers, in accordance with marijuana's status as a Schedule I drug under the Controlled Substances Act, or whether to relax federal marijuana prohibition enough to permit the medicinal use of botanical cannabis 2 products when recommended by a physician, especially in those states that have created medical marijuana programs under state law.

The first action on medical marijuana in the current Congress occurred on April 18, 2007, at markup of the Prescription Drug User Fee Act (S. 1082). The Senate Committee on Health, Education, Labor, and Pensions adopted an amendment requiring "that State-legalized medical marijuana be subject to the full regulatory requirements of the Food and Drug Administration." Intended to squelch the medical use of cannabis products that has been approved by the voters or legislatures of 12 states since 1996, the actual effect of this amendment, if signed into law, is not entirely clear and may be subject to legal interpretation, as discussed below.

Bills with the opposite intent — to allow patients who appear to benefit from medical cannabis to use it in accordance with the various state regulatory schemes that have been created — have been introduced in recent Congresses and are expected to be reintroduced in the 1 10th Congress. These include the States' Rights to Medical Marijuana Act, which would move marijuana from Schedule I to Schedule II of the Controlled Substances Act and make it available under federal law for medical use in the states with medical marijuana programs, and the Steve McWilliams Truth in Trials Act, which would make it possible for defendants in federal court to reveal to juries that their marijuana activity was medically related and legal under state law.

The Hinchey-Rohrabacher amendment, which would prohibit the use of federal funds to arrest and prosecute medical marijuana patients and providers whose activities are permitted by the laws of their states, was debated on the floor of the House on July 25, 2007, and rejected by a vote of 165 to 262. This and other congressional actions relating to the issue of medical marijuana are discussed below in greater detail.

BACKGROUND: MEDICAL MARIJUANA PRIOR TO 1937

The Cannabis sativa plant has been used for healing purposes throughout history. According to written records from China and India, the use of marijuana to treat a wide range of ailments goes back more than 2,000 years. Ancient texts from Africa, the Middle East, classical Greece, and the Roman Empire also describe the use of cannabis to treat disease.

For most of American history, growing and using marijuana was legal under both federal law and the laws of the individual states. By the 1840s, marijuana's therapeutic potential began to be recognized by some U.S. physicians. From 1850 to 1941 cannabis was included in the United States Pharmacopoeia as a recognized medicinal. [3] By the end of 1936, however, all 48 states had enacted laws to regulate marijuana. [4] Its decline in medicine was hastened by the development of aspirin, morphine, and then other opium-derived drugs, all of which helped to replace marijuana in the treatment of pain and other medical conditions in Western medicine. [5]

FEDERAL MEDICAL MARIJUANA POLICY

All three branches of the federal government play an important role in formulating federal policy on medical marijuana. Significant actions of each branch are highlighted here, beginning with the legislative branch.

Congressional Actions

The Marihuana [6] Tax Act of 1937. Spurred by spectacular accounts of marijuana's harmful effects on its users, by the drug's alleged connection to violent crime, and by a perception that state and local efforts to bring use of the drug under control were not working, Congress enacted the Marihuana Tax Act of 1937. [7] Promoted by Harry Anslinger, Commissioner of the recently established Federal Bureau of Narcotics, the act imposed registration and reporting requirements and a tax on the growers, sellers, and buyers of marijuana. Although the act did not prohibit marijuana outright, its effect was the same. (Because marijuana was not included in the Harrison Narcotics Act in 1914, [8] the Marihuana Tax Act was the federal government's first attempt to regulate marijuana.)

Dr. William C. Woodward, legislative counsel of the American Medical Association (AMA), opposed the measure. In oral testimony before the House Ways and Means Committee, he stated that "there are evidently potentialities in the drug that should not be shut off by adverse legislation. The medical profession and pharmacologists should be left to develop the use of this drug as they see fit." [9] Two months later, in a letter to the Senate Finance Committee, he again argued against the act:

> There is no evidence, however, that the medicinal use of these drugs ["cannabis and its preparations and derivatives"] has caused or is causing cannabis addiction. As remedial agents they are used to an inconsiderable extent, and the obvious purpose and effect of this bill is to impose so many restrictions on their medicinal use as to prevent such use altogether. Since the medicinal use of cannabis has not caused and is not causing addiction, the prevention of the use of the drug for medicinal purposes can accomplish no good end whatsoever. How far it may serve to deprive the public of the benefits of a drug that on further research may prove to be of substantial value, it is impossible to foresee. [10]

Despite the AMA's opposition, the Marihuana Tax Act was approved, causing all medicinal products containing marijuana to be withdrawn from the market and leading to marijuana's removal, in 1941, from The National Formulary and the United States Pharmacopoeia, in which it had been listed for almost a century.

Controlled Substances Act (1970). With increasing use of marijuana and other street drugs during the 1960s, notably by college and high school students, federal drug-control laws came under scrutiny. In July 1969, President Nixon asked Congress to enact legislation to combat rising levels of drug use. [11] Hearings were held, different proposals were considered, and House and Senate conferees filed a conference report in October 1970. [12] The report was quickly adopted by voice vote in both chambers and was signed into law as the Comprehensive Drug Abuse Prevention and Control Act of 1970 (P.L. 91-513).

Included in the new law was the Controlled Substances Act (CSA), [13] which placed marijuana and its derivatives in Schedule I, the most restrictive of five categories. Schedule I substances have "a high potential for abuse," "no currently accepted medical use in treatment in the United States," and "a lack of accepted safety [standards] for use of the drug ... under medical supervision." [14] Other drugs used recreationally at the time also became Schedule I substances. These included heroin, LSD, mescaline, peyote, and psilocybin. Drugs of abuse with recognized medical uses — such as opium, cocaine, and amphetamine — were assigned to Schedules II through V, depending on their potential for abuse. [15] Despite its placement in Schedule I, marijuana use increased, as did the number of health-care professionals and their patients who believed in the plant's therapeutic value.

The CSA does not distinguish between the medical and recreational use of marijuana. Under federal statute, simple possession of marijuana for personal use, a misdemeanor, can bring up to one year in federal prison and up to a $100,000 fine for a first offense. [16] Growing marijuana is considered manufacturing a controlled substance, a felony. [17] A single plant can bring an individual up to five years in federal prison and up to a $250,000 fine for a first offense. [18]

The CSA is not preempted by state medical marijuana laws, under the federal system of government, nor are state medical marijuana laws preempted by the CSA. States can statutorily create a medical use exception for botanical cannabis and its derivatives under their own, state-level controlled substance laws. At the same time, federal agents can investigate, arrest, and prosecute medical marijuana patients, caregivers, and providers in accordance with the federal Controlled Substances Act, even in those states where medical marijuana programs operate in accordance with state law.

Anti-Medical Marijuana Legislation in the 105th Congress (1998). In September 1998, the House debated and passed a resolution (H.J.Res. 117) declaring that Congress supports the existing federal drug approval process for determining whether any drug, including marijuana, is safe and effective and opposes efforts to circumvent this process by legalizing marijuana, or any other Schedule I drug, for medicinal use without valid scientific evidence and without approval of the Food and Drug Administration (FDA). With the Senate not acting on the resolution and adjournment approaching, this language was incorporated into the FY1999 omnibus appropriations act under the heading "Not Legalizing Marijuana for Medicinal Use." [19]

In a separate amendment to the same act, Congress prevented the District of Columbia government from counting ballots of a 1998 voter-approved initiative that would have allowed the medical use of marijuana by persons suffering from serious diseases, including cancer and HIV infection. [20] The amendment was challenged and overturned in District Court, the ballots were counted, and the measure passed 69% to 31%. Nevertheless, despite further court challenges, Congress continues to prohibit implementation of the initiative.[21]

The Hinchey-Rohrabacher Amendment (2003-2007). [22] In the first session of the 108th Congress, in response to federal Drug Enforcement Administration (DEA) raids on medical cannabis users and providers in California and other states that had approved the medical use of marijuana if recommended by a physician, Representatives Hinchey and Rohrabacher offered a bipartisan amendment to the FY2004 Commerce, Justice, State appropriations bill (H.R. 2799). The amendment would have prevented the Justice Department from using appropriated funds to interfere with the implementation of medical cannabis laws in the nine states that had approved such use. The amendment was debated on the floor of the House on July 22, 2003. When brought to a vote on the following day, it was defeated 152 to 273 (61 votes short of passage). [23]

The amendment was offered again in the second session of the 108th Congress. It was debated on the House floor on July 7, 2004, during consideration of H.R. 4754, the Commerce, Justice, State appropriations bill for FY2005. This time it would have applied to 10 states, with the recent addition of Vermont to the list of states that had approved the use of medical cannabis. It was again defeated by a similar margin, 148 to 268 (61 votes short of passage). [24]

The amendment was voted on again in the first session of the 109th Congress and was again defeated, 16 1-264 (52 votes short of passage), on June 15, 2005. During floor debate on H.R. 2862, the FY2006 Science, State, Justice, Commerce appropriations bill, a Member stated in support of the amendment that her now-deceased mother had used marijuana to treat her glaucoma. Opponents of the amendment argued, among other things, that its passage would undermine efforts to convince young people that marijuana is a dangerous drug. [25]

Despite an extensive pre-vote lobbying effort by supporters, the amendment gained only two votes in its favor over the previous year when it was debated and defeated, 163 to 259 (49 votes short of passage), on June 28, 2006. [26] The bill under consideration this time was H.R. 5672, the FY2007 Science, State, Justice, Commerce appropriations bill.

In the first session of the 1 10th Congress, on July 25, 2007, the amendment was proposed to H.R. 3093, the Commerce, Justice, Science appropriations bill for FY2008. It was debated on the House floor for the fifth time in as many years and was again rejected, 165 to 262 (49 votes short of passage). The amendment's supporters framed it as a states' rights issue:

> A vote "yes" on Hinchey-Rohrabacher is a vote to respect the intent of our Founding Fathers and respect the rights of our people at the State level to make the criminal law under which they and their families will live. It reinforces rules surrounding the patient-doctor relationship, and it is in contrast to emotional posturing and Federal power grabs and bureaucratic arrogance, which is really at the heart of the opposition. [27]

Opponents argued that smoked marijuana is not a safe and effective medicine and that it sends the wrong message to young people. The amendment is expected to be offered again as an ongoing measure of sentiment in the House for marijuana law reform.

Medical Marijuana Bills in the 1 09th Congress (2005). Bills have been introduced in recent Congresses to allow patients who appear to benefit from medical cannabis to use it in accordance with the various regulatory schemes that have been approved, since 1996, by the voters or legislatures of 12 states. This legislative activity continued in the 109th Congress.

The States' Rights to Medical Marijuana Act (H.R. 2087/Frank) would have transferred marijuana from Schedule I to Schedule II of the Controlled Substances Act. It also would have provided that, in states in which marijuana may legally be prescribed or recommended by a physician for medical use under state law, no provisions of the Controlled Substances Act or the Federal Food, Drug, and Cosmetic Act could prohibit or otherwise restrict a physician from prescribing or recommending marijuana for medical use, an individual from obtaining and using marijuana if prescribed or recommended by a physician for medical use, a pharmacy from obtaining and holding marijuana for such a prescription or recommendation, or an entity established by a state from producing and distributing marijuana for such a prescription or recommendation. Versions of this bill have been introduced in every Congress since the 105th in 1997 but have not seen action beyond the committee referral process.

Medical marijuana defendants in federal court are not permitted to introduce evidence showing that their marijuana-related activities were undertaken for a valid medical purpose under state law. The Steve McWilliams Truth in Trials Act (H.R. 4272/Farr) would have amended the Controlled Substances Act to provide an affirmative defense for the medical use of marijuana in accordance with the laws of the various states. First introduced in the 1 08th Congress, this version of the bill was named for a Californian who took his own life while awaiting federal sentencing for marijuana trafficking. At his trial, the jurors were not informed that he was actually providing marijuana to seriously ill patients in San Diego in compliance with state law. The bill also would have limited the authority of federal agents to seize marijuana authorized for medical use under state law and would have provided for the retention and return of seized plants pending resolution of a case involving medical marijuana.

Neither bill saw action beyond the committee referral process.

Legislative Activity in the 11 0th Congress. The first action on medical marijuana in the current Congress occurred during consideration of legislation to reauthorize existing FDA programs and expand the agency's authority to ensure the safety of prescription drugs, medical devices, and biologics. On April 18, 2007, at markup of the Prescription Drug User Fee Act (S. 1082), the Senate Committee on Health, Education, Labor, and Pensions adopted, in an 11-9 vote, an amendment offered by Senator Coburn designed to shut down state medical marijuana programs. The amendment stated:

> The Secretary of Health and Human Services shall require that State-legalized medical marijuana be subject to the full regulatory requirements of the Food and Drug Administration, including a risk evaluation and mitigation strategy and all other requirements of the Federal Food, Drug, and Cosmetic Act regarding safe and effective reviews, approval, sale, marketing, and use of pharmaceuticals.

Herbal cannabis products are not, in fact, being marketed in the United States as pharmaceuticals, nor are they being developed as investigational new drugs due largely to federal restrictions on marijuana research. Because of this and other possibly complicating factors, the validity and actual effect of this amendment, if signed into law, were unclear and would have been subject to legal interpretation and judicial review. [28] The bill cleared the Senate and was sent to the House on May 9. The Coburn Amendment, however, was not included in the version of the

FDA amendments act (H.R. 2900) that was approved by Congress and enacted into law (P.L. 110-85) on September 27, 2007.

In another action on medical marijuana, the House Judiciary Subcommittee on Crime, Terrorism, and Homeland Security held an oversight hearing on DEA's regulation of medicine on July 12, 2007. A DEA official testified that his agency would "continue to enforce the law as it stands and to investigate, indict, and arrest those who use the color of state law to possess and sell marijuana." A California medicinal cannabis patient and provider stated, "The well-being of thousands of seriously ill Americans backed by the opinion of the vast majority of their countrymen demands that medical marijuana be freed from federal interference." In his introduction of the patient, the subcommittee chairman observed, "Even if the law technically gives DEA the authority to investigate medical marijuana users, it is worth questioning whether targeting gravely ill people is the best use of federal resources."

Two weeks later, on July 25, the whole House decided to continue to use federal resources against medical marijuana users when it rejected the Hinchey-Rohrabacher amendment, 165-262, as described above.

In the second session of the 1 10th Congress, on April 17, 2008, Representative Frank introduced H.R. 5842, the Medical Marijuana Patient Protection Act, to provide for the medical use of marijuana in accordance with the laws of the various states. Introduced with four original co-sponsors — Representatives Farr, Hinchey, Paul, and Rohrabacher — the bill would move marijuana from schedule I to schedule II of the CSA and would, within states with medical marijuana programs, permit

- a physician to prescribe or recommend marijuana for medical use;
- an authorized patient to obtain, possess, transport, manufacture, or use marijuana;
- an authorized individual to obtain, possess, transport, or manufacture marijuana for an authorized patient; and
- a pharmacy or other authorized entity to distribute medical marijuana to authorized patients.

No provision of the Controlled Substances Act or the Federal Food, Drug, and Cosmetic Act would be allowed to prohibit or otherwise restrict these activities in states that have adopted medical marijuana programs. Also, the bill would not affect any federal, state, or local law regulating or prohibiting smoking in public. Although differently worded, H.R. 5842 has the same intent as the States' Rights to Medical Marijuana Act, versions of which have been introduced in every

Congress since the 105th in 1997. The bill was referred to the House Committee on Energy and Commerce.

In his introductory statement, Representative Frank said, "When doctors recommend the use of marijuana for their patients and states are willing to permit it, I think it's wrong for the federal government to subject either the doctors or the patients to criminal prosecution." [29]

Executive Branch Actions and Policies

IND Compassionate Access Program (1978). In 1975, a Washington, DC, resident was arrested for growing marijuana to treat his glaucoma. He won his case by using the medical necessity defense, [30] forcing the government to find a way to provide him with his medicine. In 1978, FDA created the Investigational New Drug (IND) Compassionate Access Program, [31] allowing patients whose serious medical conditions could be relieved only by marijuana to apply for and receive marijuana from the federal government. Over the next 14 years, other patients, less than 100 in total, were admitted to the program for conditions including chemotherapy-induced nausea and vomiting (emesis), glaucoma, spasticity, and weight loss. Then, in 1992, in response to a large number of applications from AIDS patients who sought to use medical cannabis to increase appetite and reverse wasting disease, the George H.W. Bush Administration closed the program to all new applicants. Several previously approved patients remain in the program today and continue to receive their monthly supply of government-grown medical marijuana.

Approval of Marinol (1985). Made by Unimed, Marinol is the trade name for dronabinol, a synthetic form of delta-9-tetrahydrocannabinol (THC), one of the principal psychoactive components of botanical marijuana. It was approved in May 1985 for nausea and vomiting associated with cancer chemotherapy in patients who fail to respond to conventional antiemetic treatments. In December 1992, it was approved by FDA for the treatment of anorexia associated with weight loss in patients with AIDS. Marketed as a capsule, Marinol was originally placed in Schedule II. [32] In July 1999, in response to a rescheduling petition from Unimed, it was moved administratively by DEA to Schedule III to make it more widely available to patients. [33] The rescheduling was granted after a review by DEA and the Department of Health and Human Services found little evidence of illicit abuse of the drug. In Schedule III, Marinol is now subject to fewer regulatory controls and lesser criminal sanctions for illicit use.

Administrative Law Judge Ruling to Reschedule Marijuana (1988). Congressional passage of the Controlled Substances Act in 1970 and its placement of marijuana in Schedule I provoked controversy at the time because it strengthened the federal policy of marijuana prohibition and forced medical marijuana users to buy marijuana of uncertain quality on the black market at inflated prices, subjecting them to fines, arrest, court costs, property forfeiture, incarceration, probation, and criminal records. The new bureaucratic controls on Schedule I substances were also criticized because they would impede research on marijuana's therapeutic potential, thereby making its evaluation and rescheduling through the normal drug approval process unlikely.

These concerns prompted a citizens' petition to the Bureau of Narcotics and Dangerous Drugs (BNDD) in 1972 to reschedule marijuana and make it available by prescription. The petition was summarily rejected. [34] This led to a long succession of appeals, hearing requests, and various court proceedings. Finally, in 1988, after extensive public hearings on marijuana's medicinal value, Francis L. Young, the chief administrative law judge of the Drug Enforcement Administration (the BNDD's successor agency), ruled on the petition, stating that "Marijuana, in its natural form, is one of the safest therapeutically active substances known to man." [35] Judge Young also wrote:

> The evidence in this record clearly shows that marijuana has been accepted as capable of relieving the distress of great numbers of very ill people, and doing so with safety under medical supervision. It would be unreasonable, arbitrary and capricious for DEA to continue to stand between those sufferers and the benefits of this substance in light of the evidence in this record.

Judge Young found that "the provisions of the [Controlled Substances] Act permit and require the transfer of marijuana from schedule I to schedule II," which would recognize its medicinal value and permit doctors to prescribe it. The judge's nonbinding findings and recommendation were soon rejected by the DEA Administrator because "marijuana has not been demonstrated as suitable for use as a medicine."36 Subsequent rescheduling petitions also have been rejected, and marijuana remains a Schedule I substance.

NIH-Sponsored Workshop (1997). NIH convened a scientific panel on medical marijuana composed of eight nonfederal experts in fields such as cancer treatment, infectious diseases, neurology, and ophthalmology. Over a two-day period in February, they analyzed available scientific information on the medical uses of marijuana and concluded that "in order to evaluate various hypotheses concerning the potential utility of marijuana in various therapeutic areas, more and better studies would be needed." Research would be justified, according to the panel, into certain conditions or diseases such as pain, neurological and movement disorders, nausea of patients undergoing chemotherapy for cancer, loss of appetite and weight related to AIDS, and glaucoma.37

Institute of Medicine Report (1999). In January 1997, shortly after passage of the California and Arizona medical marijuana initiatives, the Director of the Office of National Drug Control Policy (the federal drug czar) commissioned the Institute of Medicine (IOM) of the National Academy of Sciences to review the scientific evidence on the potential health benefits and risks of marijuana and its constituent cannabinoids. Begun in August 1997, IOM's 257-page report, Marijuana and Medicine: Assessing the Science Base, was released in March 1999.38 A review of all existing studies of the therapeutic value of cannabis, the IOM Report was also based on public hearings and consultations held around the country with biomedical and social scientists and concerned citizens.

For the most part, the IOM Report straddled the fence and provided sound bites for both sides of the medical marijuana debate. For example, "Until a nonsmoked rapid-onset cannabinoid drug delivery system becomes available, we acknowledge that there is no clear alternative for people suffering from chronic conditions that might be relieved by smoking marijuana, such as pain or AIDS-wasting" (p. 179) and "Smoked marijuana is unlikely to be a safe medication for any chronic medical condition" (p. 126). For another example, "There is no conclusive evidence that marijuana causes cancer in humans, including cancers usually related to tobacco use" (p. 119) and "Numerous studies suggest that marijuana smoke is an important risk factor in the development of respiratory disease" (p. 127).

The IOM Report did find more potential promise in synthetic cannabinoid drugs than in smoked marijuana (p. 177):

> The accumulated data suggest a variety of indications, particularly for pain relief, antiemesis, and appetite stimulation. For patients such as those with AIDS or who are undergoing chemotherapy, and who suffer simultaneously from severe pain, nausea, and appetite loss, cannabinoid drugs might offer broad-spectrum relief not found in any other single medication.

In general, the report emphasized the need for well-formulated, scientific research into the therapeutic effects of marijuana and its cannabinoid components on patients with specific disease conditions. To this end, the report recommended that clinical trials be conducted with the goal of developing safe delivery systems.

Denial of Petition to Reschedule Marijuana (2001). In response to a citizen's petition to reschedule marijuana submitted to the DEA in 1995, DEA asked the Department of Health and Human Services (HHS) for a scientific and medical evaluation of the abuse potential of marijuana and a scheduling recommendation. HHS concluded that marijuana has a high potential for abuse, no currently accepted medical use in treatment in the United States, and a lack of accepted safety for use under medical supervision. HHS therefore recommended that marijuana remain in Schedule I. In a letter to the petitioner dated March 20, 2001, DEA denied the petition. [39]

FDA Statement That Smoked Marijuana Is Not Medicine (2006). On April 20, 2006, the FDA issued an interagency advisory restating the federal government's position that "smoked marijuana is harmful" and has not been approved "for any condition or disease indication." The one-page announcement did not refer to new research findings. Instead, it was based on a "past evaluation" by several agencies within HHS that "concluded that no sound scientific studies supported medical use of marijuana for treatment in the United States, and no animal or human data supported the safety or efficacy of marijuana for general medical use." [40]

Media reaction to this pronouncement was largely negative, asserting that the FDA position on medical marijuana was motivated by politics, not science, and ignored the findings of the 1999 Institute of Medicine Report. [41] In Congress, 24 House Members, led by Representative Hinchey, sent a letter to the FDA acting commissioner requesting the scientific evidence behind the agency's evaluation of the medical efficacy of marijuana and citing the FDA's IND Compassionate Access Program as "an example of how the FDA could allow for the legal use of a drug, such as medical marijuana, without going through the 'well-controlled' series of steps that other drugs have to go through if there is a compassionate need." [42]

Administrative Law Judge Ruling to Grow Research Marijuana (2007). Since 1968, the only source of marijuana available for scientific research in the United States has been tightly controlled by the federal government. Grown at the University of Mississippi under a contract administered by the National Institute on Drug Abuse, the marijuana is difficult to obtain even by scientists whose research protocols have been approved by the FDA. Not only is the federal supply of marijuana largely inaccessible, but researchers also complain that it does not meet the needs of research due to its inferior quality and lack of multiple strains. [43] Other Schedule I substances — such as LSD, heroin, and MDMA (Ecstasy) — can be provided legally by private U.S. laboratories or imported from abroad for research purposes, with federal permission. Only marijuana is limited to a single, federally controlled provider.

In response to this situation, Dr. Lyle Craker, a professor of plant biology and director of the medicinal plant program at the University of Massachusetts at Amherst, applied in 2001 for a DEA license to cultivate research-grade marijuana. The application was filed in association with the Multidisciplinary Association for Psychedelic Studies (MAPS), a nonprofit drug research organization headed by Dr. Rick Doblin, whose stated goal is

> to break the government's monopoly on the supply of marijuana that can be used in FDA-approved research, thereby creating the proper conditions for a $5 million, 5 year drug development effort designed to transform smoked and/or vaporized marijuana into an FDA-approved prescription medicine. [44]

After being sued for "unreasonable delay" in the DC Circuit Court of Appeals, the DEA rejected the Craker/MAPS application in December 2004 as not consistent with the public interest. Upon appeal, nine days of hearings were held over a five- month period in 2005, at which researchers testified that their requests for marijuana had been rejected, making it impossible to conduct their FDA-approved research. On February 12, 2007, DEA's Administrative Law Judge Mary Ellen Bittner found that "an inadequate supply" of marijuana is available for research and ruled that it "would be in the public interest" to allow Dr. Craker to create the proposed marijuana production facility. [45] The ruling, however, is nonbinding, and a decision by the DEA Administrator on whether to accept or reject the Craker decision is pending.

DEA Enforcement Actions Against Medical Marijuana Providers. Most arrests in the United States for marijuana possession are made by state and local police, not the DEA. This means that patients and their caregivers in the states that permit medical marijuana mostly go unprosecuted, because their own state's marijuana prohibition laws do not apply to them and because federal law is not usually enforced against them.

Federal agents do, however, move against medical cannabis growers and distributors in states with medical marijuana programs. In recent years, DEA agents have conducted many raids of medical marijuana dispensaries, especially in California, where the law states that marijuana providers can receive "reasonable compensation" on a nonprofit basis. The DEA does not provide statistics on its moves against medical marijuana outlets because the agency does not distinguish between criminal, non-medical marijuana trafficking organizations and locally licensed storefront dispensaries that are legal under state law. They are all felony criminal operations under the Controlled Substances Act. As a practical matter, however, the DEA reportedly targets larger, for-profit medical marijuana providers who are engaged in "nothing more than high-stakes drug dealing, complete with the same high-rolling lifestyles." [46] A few high-profile medical marijuana patients are also being prosecuted under federal law. [47]

In July 2007, DEA's Los Angeles Field Division Office introduced a new enforcement tactic against medical marijuana dispensaries in the city when it sent letters to the owners and managers of buildings in which medical marijuana facilities are operating. The letters threaten the property owners and managers with up to 20 years in federal prison for violating the so-called "crack house statute," a provision of the CSA enacted in 1986 that made it a federal offense to "knowingly and intentionally rent, lease, or make available for use, with or without compensation, [a] building, room, or enclosure for the purpose of unlawfully manufacturing, storing, distributing, or using a controlled substance." [48] The DEA letters also threaten the landlords with seizure of their property under the CSA's asset forfeiture provisions. [49]

In response, L.A. City Council members wrote a letter to DEA Administrator Karen Tandy in Washington urging her to abandon this tactic and allow them to continue work on an ordinance to regulate medical cannabis facilities "without federal interference." They also unanimously approved a resolution endorsing the Hinchey-Rohrabacher amendment, which would prohibit such DEA actions and which was about to be debated in the House, as discussed above. An editorial in the Los Angeles Times called the DEA threats to landlords a "deplorable new bullying tactic." [50]

In subsequent months, DEA expanded this enforcement mechanism to other parts of California, including the Bay Area. In one lawsuit challenging the right of landlords to evict marijuana dispensaries, a Los Angeles County Superior Court judge ruled, in April 2008, that federal law preempts California's Compassionate Use Act. If the ruling is affirmed on appeal, it would threaten the future of medical marijuana in California and elsewhere.

DEA's actions against medical marijuana growing and distribution operations have provoked other lawsuits. In April 2003, for example, the city and county of Santa Cruz, CA, along with seven medical marijuana patients, filed a lawsuit in San Jose federal district court in response to DEA's earlier raid on the Wo/Men's Alliance for Medical Marijuana (WAMM). The court granted the plaintiffs' motion for a preliminary injunction, thereby allowing WAMM to resume growing and producing marijuana medications for its approximately 250 member-patients with serious illnesses, pending the final outcome of the case. [51] The suit is said to be the first court challenge brought by a local government against the federal war on drugs.

Medical Cannabis in the Courts: Major Cases

Because Congress and the executive branch have not acted to permit seriously ill Americans to use botanical marijuana medicinally, the issue has been considered by the judicial branch, with mixed results. Three significant cases have been decided so far, and other court challenges are moving through the judicial pipeline. [52]

U.S. v. Oakland Cannabis Buyers' Cooperative (2001). The U.S. Department of Justice filed a civil suit in January 1998 to close six medical marijuana distribution centers in northern California. A U.S. district court judge issued a temporary injunction to close the centers, pending the outcome of the case. The Oakland Cannabis Buyers' Cooperative fought the injunction but was eventually forced to cease operations and appealed to the Ninth Circuit Court of Appeals. At issue was whether a medical marijuana distributor can use a medical necessity defense against federal marijuana distribution charges. [53]

The Ninth Circuit's decision in September 1999 found, 3-0, that medical necessity is a valid defense against federal marijuana trafficking charges if a trial court finds that the patients to whom the marijuana was distributed are seriously ill, face imminent harm without marijuana, and have no effective legal alternatives. [54] The Justice Department appealed to the Supreme Court.

The Supreme Court held, 8-0, that "a medical necessity exception for marijuana is at odds with the terms of the Controlled Substances Act" because "its provisions leave no doubt that the defense is unavailable." [55] This decision had no effect on state medical marijuana laws, which continued to protect patients and primary caregivers from arrest by state and local law enforcement agents in the states with medical marijuana programs.

Conant v. Walters (2002). After the 1996 passage of California's medical marijuana initiative, the Clinton Administration threatened to investigate doctors and revoke their licenses to prescribe controlled substances and participate in Medicaid and Medicare if they recommended medical marijuana to patients under the new state law. A group of California physicians and patients filed suit in federal court, early in 1997, claiming a constitutional free-speech right, in the context of the doctor- patient relationship, to discuss the potential risks and benefits of the medical use of cannabis. A preliminary injunction, issued in April 1997, prohibited federal officials from threatening or punishing physicians for recommending marijuana to patients suffering from HIV/AIDS, cancer, glaucoma, or seizures or muscle spasms associated with a chronic, debilitating condition. [56] The court subsequently made the injunction permanent in an unpublished opinion.

On appeal, the Ninth Circuit affirmed, in a 3-0 decision, the district court's order entering a permanent injunction. The federal government, the opinion states, "may not initiate an investigation of a physician solely on the basis of a recommendation of marijuana within a bona fide doctor-patient relationship, unless the government in good faith believes that it has substantial evidence of criminal conduct." [57] The Bush Administration appealed, but the Supreme Court refused to take the case.

Gonzales v. Raich (2005). In response to DEA agents' destruction of their medical marijuana plants, two patients and two caregivers in California brought suit. They argued that applying the Controlled Substances Act to a situation in which medical marijuana was being grown and consumed locally for no remuneration in accordance with state law exceeded Congress's constitutional authority under the Commerce Clause, which allows the federal government to regulate interstate commerce. In December 2003, the Ninth Circuit Court of Appeals in San Francisco agreed, ruling 2-1 that states are free to adopt medical marijuana laws so long as the marijuana is not sold, transported across state lines, or used for nonmedical purposes. [58] Federal appeal sent the case to the Supreme Court.

The issue before the Supreme Court was whether the Controlled Substances Act, when applied to the intrastate cultivation and possession of marijuana for personal use under state law, exceeds Congress's power under the Commerce Clause. The Supreme Court, in June 2005, reversed the Ninth Circuit's decision and held, in a 6-3 decision, that Congress's power to regulate commerce extends to purely local activities that are "part of an economic class of activities that have a substantial effect on interstate commerce." [59]

Raich does not invalidate state medical marijuana laws. The decision does mean, however, that DEA may continue to enforce the CSA against medical marijuana patients and their caregivers, even in states with medical marijuana programs.

Although Raich was not about the efficacy of medical marijuana or its listing in Schedule I, the majority opinion stated in a footnote: "We acknowledge that evidence proffered by respondents in this case regarding the effective medical uses for marijuana, if found credible after trial, would cast serious doubt on the accuracy of the findings that require marijuana to be listed in Schedule I." [60] The majority opinion, in closing, notes that in the absence of judicial relief for medical marijuana users there remains "the democratic process, in which the voices of voters allied with these respondents may one day be heard in the halls of Congress." [61]

Thus, the Supreme Court reminds that Congress has the power to reschedule marijuana, thereby recognizing that it has accepted medical use in treatment in the United States. Congress, however, does not appear likely to do so. Neither does the executive branch, which could reschedule marijuana through regulatory procedures authorized by the Controlled Substances Act. In the meantime, actions taken by state and local governments continue to raise the issue, as discussed below.

Americans for Safe Access (ASA) Lawsuit Against HHS. The federal Data Quality Act of 2001 (DQA) requires the issuance of guidelines "for ensuring and maximizing the quality, objectivity, utility, and integrity of information (including statistical information) disseminated by Federal agencies" and allows "affected persons to seek and obtain correction of information maintained and disseminated by the agency that does not comply with the guidelines." [62]

In October 2004, Americans for Safe Access (ASA), a California-based patient advocacy group, formally petitioned HHS, under the DQA, to correct four erroneous statements about medical marijuana made by HHS in its 2001 denial of the marijuana rescheduling petition discussed above. Specifically, ASA requested that "there have been no studies that have scientifically assessed the efficacy of marijuana for any medical condition" be replaced with "[a]dequate and well-recognized studies show the efficacy of marijuana in the treatment of nausea, loss of appetite, pain and spasticity"; that "it is clear that there is not a consensus of medical opinion concerning medical applications of marijuana" be replaced with "[t]here is substantial consensus among experts in the relevant disciplines that marijuana is effective in treating nausea, loss of appetite, pain and spasticity. It is accepted as medicine by qualified experts"; that "complete scientific analysis of all the chemical components found in marijuana has not been conducted" be replaced with "[t]he chemistry of marijuana is known and reproducible"; and that "marijuana has no currently accepted medical use in treatment in the United States" be replaced with "[m]arijuana has a currently accepted use in treatment in the United States." The petition claimed that "HHS's statements about the lack of medical usefulness of marijuana harms these individuals [ill persons across the United States] in that it contributes to denying them access to medicine which will alleviate their suffering." [63]

Were HHS to accept the ASA petition, the revised statements would set the preconditions for placing marijuana in a schedule other than I. HHS denied the petition in 2005 and rejected ASA's subsequent appeal in 2006 on just those grounds: that HHS is already in the process of reviewing a rescheduling petition submitted to DEA in October 2002 and will be evaluating all of the publicly available peer- reviewed literature on the medicinal efficacy of marijuana in that context. In response, in February 2007, ASA filed suit in U.S. District Court for the Northern District of California to force HHS to change the four statements, which the organization believes are not science-based. The case is pending.

STATE AND LOCAL REFERENDA AND LEGISLATION

In the face of federal intransigence on the issue, advocates of medical marijuana have turned to the states in a largely successful effort, wherever it has been attempted, to enact laws that enable patients to obtain and use botanical marijuana therapeutically in a legal and regulated manner, even though such activity remains illegal under federal law.

States Allowing Use of Medical Marijuana [64]

Twelve states, covering about 22% of the U.S. population, have enacted laws to allow the use of cannabis for medical purposes. [65] These states have removed state- level criminal penalties for the cultivation, possession, and use of medical marijuana, if such use has been recommended by a medical doctor.

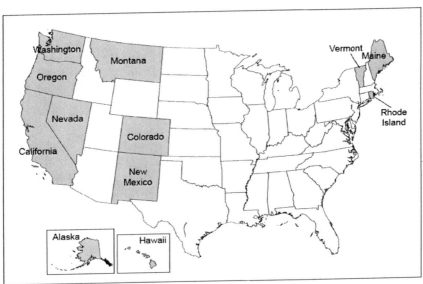

Source: Map Resources. Adapted by CRS.

Figure 1. States With Medical Marijuana Programs.

All of these states have in place, or are developing, programs to regulate the use of medical marijuana by approved patients. Patients in state programs (except for New Mexico) may be assisted by caregivers, persons who are authorized to help patients grow, acquire, and use the drug. Physicians in these states are immune from liability and prosecution for discussing or recommending medical cannabis to their patients in accordance with state law.

Nine of the 12 states that have legalized medical marijuana are in the West: Alaska, California, Colorado, Hawaii, Montana, Nevada, New Mexico, Oregon, and Washington. Of the 37 states outside the West, only three, all in the Northeast — Maine, Rhode Island, and Vermont — have adopted medical cannabis statutes. Hawaii, New Mexico, Rhode Island, and Vermont have the only programs initiated by acts of their state legislatures. The medical marijuana programs in the other eight states were approved by the voters in statewide referenda or ballot initiatives, beginning in 1996 with California. Since then, voters have approved medical marijuana initiatives in every state where they have appeared on the ballot with the exception of South Dakota, where a medical marijuana initiative was defeated in 2006 by 52% of the voters. Bills to create medical marijuana programs have been introduced in the legislatures of additional states — Alabama, Connecticut, Illinois, Maryland, Minnesota, New Hampshire, New Jersey, among others — and have received varying levels of consideration but have so far not been enacted.

Effective state medical marijuana laws do not attempt to overturn or otherwise violate federal laws that prohibit doctors from writing prescriptions for marijuana and pharmacies from distributing it. In the 12 states with medical marijuana programs, doctors do not actually prescribe marijuana, and the marijuana products used by patients are not distributed through pharmacies. Rather, doctors recommend marijuana to their patients, and the cannabis products are grown by patients or their caregivers, or they are obtained from cooperatives or other alternative dispensaries. The state medical marijuana programs do, however, contravene the federal prohibition of marijuana. Medical marijuana patients, their caregivers, and other marijuana providers can, therefore, be arrested by federal law enforcement agents, and they can be prosecuted under federal law.

Statistics on Medical Marijuana Users. Determining exactly how many patients use medical marijuana with state approval is difficult. According to a 2002 study published in the Journal of Cannabis Therapeutics, an estimated 30,000 California patients and another 5,000 patients in eight other states possessed a physician's recommendations to use cannabis medically. [66] More recent estimates are much higher. The New England Journal of Medicine reported in August 2005, for example, that an estimated 115,000 people have obtained marijuana recommendations from doctors in the states with programs. [67]

Although 115,000 people may be approved medical marijuana users, the number of patients who have actually registered is much lower. A July 2005 CRS telephone survey of the state programs revealed a total of 14,758 registered medical marijuana users in eight states. [68] (Maine and Washington do not maintain state registries, and Rhode Island and New Mexico had not yet passed their laws.) This number vastly understates the number of medical marijuana users, however, because California's state registry was in pilot status, with only 70 patients so far registered.

A brief description of each state's medical marijuana programs follows. The programs are discussed in the order in which they were approved by voters or passed by the state legislatures.

California (1996). Proposition 215, approved by 56% of the voters in November, removed the state's criminal penalties for medical marijuana use, possession, and cultivation by patients with the "written or oral recommendation or approval of a physician" who has determined that the patient's "health would benefit from medical marijuana." Called the Compassionate Use Act, it legalized cannabis for "the treatment of cancer, anorexia, AIDS, chronic pain, spasticity, glaucoma, arthritis, migraine, or any other illness for which marijuana provides relief." The law permits possession of an amount sufficient for the patient's "personal medical purposes." A second statute (Senate bill 420), passed in 2003, allows "reasonable compensation" for medical marijuana caregivers and says that distribution should be done on a nonprofit basis.

Oregon (1998). Voters in November removed the state's criminal penalties for use, possession, and cultivation of marijuana by patients whose physicians advise that marijuana "may mitigate the symptoms or effects" of a debilitating condition. The law, approved by 55% of Oregon voters, does not provide for distribution of cannabis but allows up to seven plants per patient (changed to 24 plants by act of the state legislature in 2005). The state registry program is supported by patient fees. (In the November 2004 election, 58% of Oregon voters rejected a measure that would have expanded the state's existing program.)

Alaska (1998). Voters in November approved a ballot measure to remove state-level criminal penalties for patients diagnosed by a physician as having a debilitating medical condition for which other approved medications were considered. The measure was approved by 58% of the voters. In 1999, the state legislature created a mandatory state registry for medical cannabis users and limited the amount a patient can legally possess to 1 ounce and six plants.

Washington (1998). Approved in November by 59% of the voters, the ballot initiative exempts from prosecution patients who meet all qualifying criteria, possess no more marijuana than is necessary for their own personal medical use (but no more than a 60-day supply), and present valid documentation to investigating law enforcement officers. The state does not issue identification cards to patients.

Maine (1999). Maine's ballot initiative, passed in November by 61% of the voters, puts the burden on the state to prove that a patient's medical use or possession is not authorized by statute. Patients with a qualifying condition, authenticated by a physician, who have been "advised" by the physician that they "might benefit" from medical cannabis, are permitted 11/4 ounces and six plants. There is no state registry of patients.

Hawaii (2000). In June, the Hawaii legislature approved a bill removing state-level criminal penalties for medical cannabis use, possession, and cultivation of up to seven plants. A physician must certify that the patient has a debilitating condition for which "the potential benefits of the medical use of marijuana would likely outweigh the health risks." This was the first state law permitting medical cannabis use that was enacted by a legislature instead of by ballot initiative.

Colorado (2000). A ballot initiative to amend the state constitution was approved by 54% of the voters in November. The amendment provides that lawful medical cannabis users must be diagnosed by a physician as having a debilitating condition and be "advised" by the physician that the patient "might benefit" from using the drug. A patient and the patient's caregiver may possess 2 usable ounces and six plants.

Nevada (2000). To amend the state constitution by ballot initiative, a proposed amendment must be approved by the voters in two separate elections. In November, 65% of Nevada voters passed for the second time an amendment to exempt medical cannabis users from prosecution. Patients who have "written documentation" from their physicians that marijuana may alleviate their health condition may register with the state Department of Agriculture and receive an identification card that exempts them from state prosecution for using medical marijuana.

Vermont (2004). In May, Vermont became the second state to legalize medical cannabis by legislative action instead of ballot initiative. Vermont patients are allowed to grow up to three marijuana plants in a locked room and to possess 2 ounces of manicured marijuana under the supervision of the Department of Public Safety, which maintains a patient registry. The law went into effect without the signature of the governor, who declined to sign it but also refused to veto it, despite pressure from Washington. A 2007 legislative act expanded eligibility for the program and increased to nine the number of plants participants may grow.

Montana (2004). In November, 62% of state voters passed Initiative 148, allowing qualifying patients to use marijuana under medical supervision. Eligible medical conditions include cancer, glaucoma, HIV/AIDS, wasting syndrome, seizures, and severe or chronic pain. A doctor must certify that the patient has a debilitating medical condition and that the benefits of using marijuana would likely outweigh the risks. The patient may grow up to six plants and possess 1 ounce of dried marijuana. The state public health department registers patients and caregivers.

Rhode Island (2006). In January, the state legislature overrode the governor's veto of a medical marijuana bill, allowing patients to possess up to 12 plants or 2 1/2 ounces to treat cancer, HIV/AIDS, and other chronic ailments. The law included a sunset provision and was set to expire on July 1, 2007, unless renewed by the legislature. The law was made permanent on June 21, 2007, after legislators voted again to override the governor's veto by a wide margin.

New Mexico (2007). Passed by the legislature and signed into law by the governor in April, the Lynn and Erin Compassionate Use Medical Marijuana Act went into effect on July 1, 2007. It requires the state's Department of Health to set rules governing the distribution of medical cannabis to state-authorized patients. Unlike other state programs, patients and their caregivers cannot grow their own marijuana; rather, it will be provided by state-licensed "cannabis production facilities."

Other State and Local Medical Marijuana Laws

Arizona (1996). Arizona's law, [69] approved by 65% of the voters in November, permits marijuana prescriptions, but there is no active program in the state because federal law prohibits doctors from prescribing marijuana. Patients cannot, therefore, obtain a valid prescription. (Other states' laws allow doctors to "recommend" rather than "prescribe.")

Maryland (2003). Maryland's General Assembly became the second state legislature, after Hawaii, to protect medical cannabis patients from the threat of jail when it approved a bill, later signed by the governor, providing that patients using marijuana preparations to treat the symptoms of illnesses such as cancer, AIDS, and Crohn's disease would be subject to no more than a $100 fine. [70] The law falls short of full legalization and does not create a medical marijuana program, but it allows for a medical necessity defense for people who use marijuana on their own for medical purposes. If patients arrested for possession in Maryland can prove in court that they use cannabis for legitimate medical needs, they escape the maximum penalty of one year in jail and a $1,000 fine.

Other State Laws. Laws favorable to medical marijuana have been enacted in 36 states since 1978. [71] Except for the state laws mentioned above, however, these laws do not currently protect medical marijuana users from state prosecution. Some laws, for example, allow patients to acquire and use cannabis through therapeutic research programs, although none of these programs has been operational since 1985, due in large part to federal opposition. Other state laws allow doctors to prescribe marijuana or allow patients to possess marijuana if it has been obtained through a prescription, but the federal Controlled Substances Act prevents these laws from being implemented. Several states have placed marijuana in a controlled drug schedule that recognizes its medical value. State legislatures continue to consider medical marijuana bills, some favorable to its use by patients, others not. In Michigan, a medical marijuana initiative will be presented to the voters on the November 2008 ballot.

District of Columbia (1998). In the nation's capital, 69% of voters approved a medical cannabis initiative to allow patients a "sufficient quantity" of marijuana to treat illness and to permit nonprofit marijuana suppliers. Congress, however, has blocked the initiative from taking effect. [72]

Local Measures. Medical cannabis measures have been adopted in several localities throughout the country. San Diego is the country's largest city to do so. One day after the Supreme Court's anti-marijuana ruling in Gonzales v. Raich was issued, Alameda County in California approved an ordinance to regulate medical marijuana dispensaries, becoming the 17th locality in the state to do so. Localities in nonmedical marijuana states have also acted. In November 2004, for example, voters in Columbia, MO, and Ann Arbor, MI, approved medical cannabis measures. Since then, four other Michigan cities, including Detroit, have done the same. Although largely symbolic, such local laws can influence the priorities of local law enforcement officers and prosecutors.

PUBLIC OPINION ON MEDICAL MARIJUANA

Voters in eight states have approved medical marijuana initiatives to protect patients from arrest under state law. Likewise, American public opinion has consistently favored access to medical marijuana by seriously ill patients. ProCon.org, a nonprofit and nonpartisan public education foundation, has identified 21 national public opinion polls that asked questions about medical marijuana from 1995 to the present. Respondents in every poll were in favor of medical marijuana by substantial margins, ranging from 60% to 85%. [73]

The Journal of the American Medical Association analyzed public opinion on the War on Drugs in a 1998 article. The authors' observations concerning public attitudes toward medical marijuana remain true today:

> While opposing the use or legalization of marijuana for recreational purposes, the public apparently does not want to deny very ill patients access to a potentially helpful drug therapy if prescribed by their physicians. The public's support of marijuana for medical purposes is conditioned by their belief that marijuana would be used only in the treatment of serious medical conditions. [74]

In public opinion polls, then, the majority of Americans appear to hold that seriously ill or terminal patients should be able to use marijuana if recommended by their doctors. Twelve state governments have created medical marijuana programs, either through ballot initiatives or the legislative process. Many other state governments, however, along with the federal government, remain opposed to the national majority in favor of medical marijuana.

ANALYSIS OF ARGUMENTS FOR AND AGAINST MEDICAL MARIJUANA

In the ongoing debate over cannabis as medicine, certain arguments are frequently made on both sides of the issue. These arguments are briefly stated below and are analyzed in turn. Equal weight is not given to both sides of every argument. Instead, the analysis is weighted according to the preponderance of evidence as currently understood. CRS takes no position on the claims or counterclaims in this debate.

What follows is an attempt to analyze objectively the claims frequently made about the role that herbal cannabis might or might not play in the treatment of certain diseases and about the possible societal consequences should its role in the practice of modern medicine be expanded beyond the places where it is now permitted under state laws.

For those interested in learning more about medical marijuana research findings, the Internet offers two useful websites. The International Association for Cannabis as Medicine (IACM), based in Germany, provides abundant information on the results of controlled clinical trials at [http://www.cannabis-med.org].

Information on peer-reviewed, double-blind studies on both animals and human subjects conducted since 1990 has been compiled by ProCon.org and is available at [http://www.medical marijuanaprocon.org].

Marijuana Is Harmful and Has No Medical Value

> Suitable and superior medicines are currently available for treatment of all symptoms alleged to be treatable by crude marijuana.
> — Brief of the Drug Free America Foundation, et al., 2004 [75]

The federal government — along with many state governments and private antidrug organizations — staunchly maintains that botanical marijuana is a dangerous drug without any legitimate medical use. Marijuana intoxication can impair a person's coordination and decision-making skills and alter behavior. Chronic marijuana smoking can adversely affect the lungs, the cardiovascular system, and possibly the immune and reproductive systems. [76]

Of course, FDA's 1985 approval of Marinol proves that the principal psychoactive ingredient of marijuana — THC — has therapeutic value. But that is not the issue in the medical marijuana debate. Botanical marijuana remains a plant substance, an herb, and its opponents say it cannot substitute for legitimate pharmaceuticals. Just because certain molecules found in marijuana might have become approved medicines, they argue, does not make the unpollinated bud of the female Cannabis sativa plant a safe and effective medicine. The Drug Free America Foundation calls the medical use of crude marijuana "a step backward to the times of potions and herbal remedies." [77]

The federal government's argument that marijuana has no medical value is straightforward. A drug, in order to meet the standard of the Controlled Substances Act as having a "currently accepted medical use in treatment in the United States," must meet a five-part test:

(1)   The drug's chemistry must be known and reproducible,
(2)   there must be adequate safety studies,
(3)   there must be adequate and well-controlled studies proving efficacy,
(4)   the drug must be accepted by qualified experts, and
(5)   the scientific evidence must be widely available. [78]

According to the DEA, botanical marijuana meets none of these requirements. First, marijuana's chemistry is neither fully known nor reproducible. Second, adequate safety studies have not been done. Third, there are no adequate, well-controlled scientific studies proving marijuana is effective for any medical condition. Fourth, marijuana is not accepted by even a significant minority of experts qualified to evaluate drugs. Fifth, published scientific evidence concluding that marijuana is safe and effective for use in humans does not exist. [79]

The same DEA Final Order that set forth the five requirements for currently accepted medical use also outlined scientific evidence that would be considered irrelevant by the DEA in establishing currently accepted medical use. These include individual case reports, clinical data collected by practitioners, studies conducted by persons not qualified by scientific training and experience to evaluate the safety and effectiveness of the substance at issue, and studies or reports so lacking in detail as to preclude responsible scientific evaluation. Such information is inadequate for experts to conclude responsibly and fairly that marijuana is safe and effective for use as medicine. [80] The DEA and other federal drug control agencies can thereby disregard medical literature and opinion that claim to show the therapeutic value of marijuana because they do not meet the government's standards of proof.

The official view of medical marijuana is complicated by the wider War on Drugs. It is difficult to disentangle the medical use of locally grown marijuana for personal use from the overall policy of marijuana prohibition, as the Supreme Court made clear in Raich. To make an exemption for medical marijuana, the Court decided, "would undermine the orderly enforcement of the entire regulatory scheme ... The notion that California law has surgically excised a discrete activity that is hermetically sealed off from the larger interstate marijuana market is a dubious proposition...." [81]

It remains the position of the federal government, then, that the Schedule I substance marijuana is harmful — not beneficial — to human health. Its use for any reason, including medicinal, should continue to be prohibited and punished. Despite signs of a more tolerant public attitude toward medical marijuana, its therapeutic benefits, if any, will continue to be officially unacknowledged and largely unrealized in the United States so long as this position prevails at the federal level.

Marijuana Effectively Treats the Symptoms of Some Diseases

[I]t cannot seriously be contested that there exists a small but significant class of individuals who suffer from painful chronic, degenerative, and terminal conditions, for whom marijuana provides uniquely effective relief.
— Brief of the Leukemia and Lymphoma Society, et al., 2004 [82]

Proponents of medical marijuana point to a large body of studies from around the world that support the therapeutic value of marijuana in treating a variety of disease-related problems, including:

- relieving nausea,
- increasing appetite,
- reducing muscle spasms and spasticity,
- relieving chronic pain,
- reducing intraocular pressure, and
- relieving anxiety. [83]

Given these properties, marijuana has been used successfully to treat the debilitating symptoms of cancer and cancer chemotherapy, [84] AIDS, multiple sclerosis, epilepsy, glaucoma, anxiety, and other serious illnesses. [85] As opponents of medical marijuana assert, existing FDA-approved pharmaceuticals for these conditions are generally more effective than marijuana. Nevertheless, as the IOM Report acknowledged, the approved medicines do not work for everyone. [86] Many medical marijuana users report trying cannabis only reluctantly and as a last resort after exhausting all other treatment modalities. A distinct subpopulation of patients now relies on whole cannabis for a degree of relief that FDA-approved synthetic drugs do not provide.

Medical cannabis proponents claim that single-cannabinoid, synthetic pharmaceuticals like Marinol are poor substitutes for the whole marijuana plant, which contains more than 400 known chemical compounds, including about 60 active cannabinoids in addition to THC. They say that scientists are a long way from knowing for sure which ones, singly or in combination, provide which therapeutic effects. Many patients have found that they benefit more from the whole plant than from any synthetically produced chemical derivative. [87] Furthermore, the natural plant can be grown easily and inexpensively, whereas Marinol and any other cannabis- based pharmaceuticals that might be developed in the future will likely be expensive — prohibitively so for some patients. [88]

In recognition of the therapeutic benefits of botanical marijuana products, various associations of health professionals have passed resolutions in support of medical cannabis. These include the American Public Health Association, the American Nurses Association, and the California Pharmacists Association. The New England Journal of Medicine has editorialized in favor of patient access to marijuana. [89] Other groups, such as the American Medical Association, are more cautious. Their position is that not enough is known about botanical marijuana and that more research is needed. [90]

The recent discovery of cannabinoid receptors in the human brain and immune system provides a biological explanation for the claimed effectiveness of marijuana in relieving multiple disease symptoms. The human body produces its own cannabis- like compounds, called endocannabinoids, that react with the body's cannabinoid receptors. Like the better known opiate receptors, the cannabinoid receptors in the brain stem and spinal cord play a role in pain control. Cannabinoid receptors, which are abundant in various parts of the human brain, also play a role in controlling the vomiting reflex, appetite, emotional responses, motor skills, and memory formation. It is the presence of these natural, endogenous cannabinoids in the human nervous and immune systems that provides the basis for the therapeutic value of marijuana and that holds the key, some scientists believe, to many promising drugs of the future. [91]

The federal government's own IND Compassionate Access Program, which has provided government-grown medical marijuana to a select group of patients since 1978, provides important evidence that marijuana has medicinal value and can be used safely. A scientist and organizer of the California medical marijuana initiative, along with two medical-doctor colleagues, has written:

> Nothing reveals the contradictions in federal policy toward marijuana more clearly than the fact that there are still eight patients in the United States who receive a tin of marijuana 'joints' (cigarettes) every month from the federal government.... These eight people can legally possess and use marijuana, at government expense and with government permission. Yet hundreds of thousands of other patients can be fined and jailed under federal law for doing exactly the same thing. [92]

Smoking Is an Improper Route of Drug Administration

> Can you think of any other untested, home-made, mind-altering medicine that you self-dose, and that uses a burning carcinogen as a delivery vehicle?
> — General Barry McCaffrey, U.S. Drug Czar, 1996-2000 [93]

That medical marijuana is smoked is probably the biggest obstacle preventing its wider acceptance. Opponents of medical marijuana argue that smoking is a poor way to take a drug, that inhaling smoke is an unprecedented drug delivery system, even though many approved medications are marketed as inhalants. DEA Administrator Karen Tandy writes:

The scientific and medical communities have determined that smoked marijuana is a health danger, not a cure. There is no medical evidence that smoking marijuana helps patients. In fact, the Food and Drug Administration (FDA) has approved no medications that are smoked, primarily because smoking is a poor way to deliver medicine. Morphine, for example has proven to be a medically valuable drug, but the FDA does not endorse smoking opium or heroin. [94]

Medical marijuana opponents argue that chronic marijuana smoking is harmful to the lungs, the cardiovascular system, and possibly the immune and reproductive systems. These claims may be overstated to help preserve marijuana prohibition. For example, neither epidemiological nor aggregate clinical data show higher rates of lung cancer in people who smoke marijuana. [95] The other alleged harms also remain unproven. Even if smoking marijuana is proven harmful, however, the immediate benefits of smoked marijuana could still outweigh the potential long-term harms — especially for terminally ill patients. [96]

The therapeutic value of smoked marijuana is supported by existing research and experience. For example, the following statements appeared in the American Medical Association's "Council on Scientific Affairs Report 10 — Medicinal Marijuana," [97] adopted by the AMA House of delegates on December 9, 1997:

- "Smoked marijuana was comparable to or more effective than oral THC [Marinol], and considerably more effective than prochlorperazine or other previous antiemetics in reducing nausea and emesis." (p. 10)
- "Anecdotal, survey, and clinical data support the view that smoked marijuana and oral THC provide symptomatic relief in some patients with spasticity associated with multiple sclerosis (MS) or trauma." (p. 13)
- "Smoked marijuana may benefit individual patients suffering from intermittent or chronic pain." (p. 15)

The IOM Report expressed concerns about smoking (p. 126): "Smoked marijuana is unlikely to be a safe medication for any chronic medical condition." Despite this concern, the IOM Report's authors were willing to recommend smoked marijuana under certain limited circumstances. For example, the report states (p. 154):

Until the development of rapid-onset antiemetic drug delivery systems, there will likely remain a subpopulation of patients for whom standard antiemetic therapy is ineffective and who suffer from debilitating emesis. It is possible that the harmful effects of smoking marijuana for a limited period of time might be outweighed by the antiemetic benefits of marijuana, at least for patients for whom standard antiemetic therapy is ineffective and who suffer from debilitating emesis. Such patients should be evaluated on a case-by-case basis and treated under close medical supervision.

The IOM Report makes another exception for terminal cancer patients (p. 159):

> Terminal cancer patients pose different issues. For those patients the medical harm associated with smoking is of little consequence. For terminal patients suffering debilitating pain or nausea and for whom all indicated medications have failed to provide relief, the medical benefits of smoked marijuana might outweigh the harm.

Smoking can actually be a preferred drug delivery system for patients whose nausea prevents them from taking anything orally. Such patients need to inhale their antiemitic drug. Other patients prefer inhaling because the drug is absorbed much more quickly through the lungs, so that the beneficial effects of the drug are felt almost at once. This rapid onset also gives patients more control over dosage. For a certain patient subpopulation, then, these advantages of inhalation may prevail over both edible marijuana preparations and pharmaceutical drugs in pill form, such as Marinol.

Moreover, medical marijuana advocates argue that there are ways to lessen the risks of smoking. Any potential problems associated with smoking, they argue, can be reduced by using higher potency marijuana, which means that less has to be inhaled to achieve the desired therapeutic effect. Furthermore, marijuana does not have to be smoked to be used as medicine. It can be cooked in various ways and eaten. [98] Like Marinol, however, taking marijuana orally can be difficult for patients suffering from nausea. Many patients are turning to vaporizers, which offer the benefits of smoking — rapid action, ease of dose titration — without having to inhale smoke. Vaporizers are devices that take advantage of the fact that cannabinoids vaporize at a lower temperature than that required for marijuana to burn. Vaporizers heat the plant matter enough for the cannabinoids to be released as vapor without having to burn the marijuana preparation. Patients can thereby inhale the beneficial cannabinoids without also having to inhale the potentially harmful by-products of marijuana combustion. [99]

Marijuana Should Be Rescheduled To Permit Medical Use

[T]he administrative law judge concludes that the provisions of the [Controlled Substances] Act permit and require the transfer of marijuana from Schedule I to Schedule II. The Judge realizes that strong emotions are aroused on both sides of any discussion concerning the use of marijuana. Nonetheless it is essential for this Agency [DEA], and its Administrator, calmly and dispassionately to review the evidence of record, correctly apply the law, and act accordingly.
— Francis L. Young, DEA Administrative Law Judge, 1988 [100]

Proponents of medical marijuana believe its placement in Schedule I of the CSA was an error from the beginning. Cannabis is one of the safest therapeutically active substances known. [101] No one has ever died of an overdose. [102] Petitions to reschedule marijuana have been received by the federal government, and rejected, ever since the original passage of the Controlled Substances Act in 1970.

Rescheduling can be accomplished administratively or it can be done by an act of Congress. Administratively, the federal Department of Health and Human Services (HHS) could find that marijuana meets sufficient standards of safety and efficacy to warrant rescheduling. Even though THC, the most prevalent cannabinoid in marijuana, was administratively moved to Schedule III in 1999, no signs exist that botanical marijuana will similarly be rescheduled by federal agency ruling anytime soon.

An act of Congress to reschedule marijuana is only slightly less likely, although such legislation has been introduced in recent Congresses including the 109th . [103] The States' Rights to Medical Marijuana Act (H.R. 2087/Frank), which would move marijuana from Schedule I to Schedule II of the Controlled Substances Act, has seen no action beyond committee referral. [104]

Schedule II substances have a high potential for abuse and may lead to severe psychological or physical dependence but have a currently accepted medical use in treatment in the United States. Cocaine, methamphetamine, morphine, and methadone are classified as Schedule II substances. Many drug policy experts and laypersons alike believe that marijuana should also reside in Schedule II.

Others think marijuana should be properly classified as a Schedule III substance, along with THC and its synthetic version, Marinol. Substances in Schedule III have less potential for abuse than the drugs in Schedules I and II, their abuse may lead to moderate or low physical dependence or high psychological dependence, and they have a currently accepted medical use in treatment in the United States.

Rescheduling seems to be supported by public opinion. A nationwide Gallup Poll conducted in March 1999 found that 73% of American adults favor "making marijuana legally available for doctors to prescribe in order to reduce pain and suffering." An AARP poll of American adults age 45 and older conducted in mid-November 2004 found that 72% agree that adults should be allowed to legally use marijuana for medical purposes if recommended by a physician. [105]

Few Members of Congress, however, publicly support the rescheduling option. The States' Rights to Medical Marijuana Act (H.R. 2087/Frank), which would move marijuana from Schedule I to Schedule II of the Controlled Substances Act, currently has 37 cosponsors.

State Medical Marijuana Laws Increase Illicit Drug Use

> The natural extension of this myth [that marijuana is good medicine] is that, if marijuana is medicine, it must also be safe for recreational use.
> — Karen P. Tandy, DEA Administrator, 2005 [106]

It is the position of the federal government that to permit the use of medical marijuana affords the drug a degree of legitimacy it does not deserve. America's youth are especially vulnerable, it is said, and state medical marijuana programs send the wrong message to our youth, many of whom do not recognize the very real dangers of marijuana.

Studies show that the use of an illicit drug is inversely proportional to the perceived harm of that drug. That is, the more harmful a drug is perceived to be, the fewer the number of people who will try it. [107] Opponents of medical marijuana argue that "surveys show that perception of harm with respect to marijuana has been dropping off annually since the renewal of the drive to legalize marijuana as medicine, which began in the early 1990s when legalization advocates first gained a significant increase in funding and began planning the state ballot initiative drive to legalize crude marijuana as medicine." [108] They point to the 1999 National Household Survey on Drug Abuse (NHSDA), which "reveals that those states which have passed medical marijuana laws have among the highest levels of past-month marijuana use, of past-month other drug use, of drug addiction, and of drug and alcohol addiction." [109]

Indeed, all 11 states that have passed medical marijuana laws ranked above the national average in the percentage of persons 12 or older reporting past-month use of marijuana in 1999, as shown in Table 3. It is at least possible, however, that this analysis confuses cause with effect. It is logical to assume that the states with the highest prevalence of marijuana usage would be more likely to approve medical marijuana programs, because the populations of those states would be more knowledgeable of marijuana's effects and more tolerant of its use.

Tables 1. States Ranked by Percentage of Youth Age 12-17 Reporting Past-Month Marijuana Use, 1999

Rank	State	%
1	Delaware	13.9
2	Massachusetts	11.9
3	Nevada	11.6
4	Montana	11.4
5	Rhode Island	10.8
6	New Hampshire	10.7
7	Alaska	10.4
8	Colorado	10.3
9	Minnesota	9.9
9	Washington	9.9
11	Oregon	9.6
	District of Columbia	9.6
12	Illinois	9.2
12	New Mexico	9.2
14	Maryland	8.8
15	Indiana	8.7
16	Connecticut	8.6
17	Vermont	8.4
18	Hawaii	8.3
18	Wisconsin	8.3
20	Michigan	7.8
20	Wyoming	7.8
22	California	7.7
23	North Dakota	7.6
	National	7.4
24	South Carolina	7.4
27	Arizona	7.3
27	Arkansas	7.3
27	New Jersey	7.3
28	Maine	7.2
29	West Virginia	7.1
31	Ohio	6.9
31	South Dakota	6.9
33	New York	6.8

Rank	State	%
33	North Carolina	6.8
34	Mississippi	6.7
37	Kansas	6.6
37	Louisiana	6.6
37	Missouri	6.6
38	Georgia	6.4
40	Oklahoma	6.3
40	Pennsylvania	6.3
41	Florida	6.2
43	Nebraska	6.1
43	Utah	6.1
45	Idaho	5.9
45	Virginia	5.9
46	Texas	5.7
47	Alabama	5.6
48	Kentucky	5.3
50	Iowa	5.2
50	Tennessee	5.2

Source: SAMHSA, Office of Applied Studies, National Household Survey on Drug Abuse, 1999, Table 3B, at [http://www.oas.samhsa.gov/ NHSDA/99 StateTabs/tables2.htm]. Rankings calculated by CRS.

It is also the case that California, the state with the largest and longest-running medical marijuana program, ranked 34th in the percentage of persons age 12-17 reporting marijuana use in the past month during the period 2002-2003, as shown in Table 2. In fact, between 1999 and 2002-2003, of the 10 states with active medical marijuana programs, five states (AK, HI, ME, MT, VT) rose in the state rankings of past-month marijuana use by 12- to 17-year-olds and five states fell (CA, CO, NV, OR, WA). [110] Of the five states that had approved medical marijuana laws before 1999 (AK, AZ, CA, OR, WA), only Alaska's ranking rose between 1999 and 2002- 2003, from 7th to 4th , with 11.08% of youth reporting past-month marijuana use in 2002-2003 compared with 10.4% in 1999. No clear patterns are apparent in the state- level data. Clearly, more important factors are at work in determining a state's prevalence of recreational marijuana use than whether the state has a medical marijuana program.

The IOM Report found no evidence for the supposition that state medical marijuana programs lead to increased use of marijuana or other drugs (pp. 6-7):

> Finally, there is a broad social concern that sanctioning the medical use of marijuana might increase its use among the general population. At this point there are no convincing data to support this concern. The existing data are

consistent with the idea that this would not be a problem if the medical use of marijuana were as closely regulated as other medications with abuse potential.... [T]his question is beyond the issues normally considered for medical uses of drugs and should not be a factor in evaluating the therapeutic potential of marijuana or cannabinoids.

Tables 2. States Ranked by Percentage of Youth Age 12-17 Reporting Past-Month Marijuana Use, 2002-2003

Rank	State	%
1	Vermont	13.32
2	Montana	12.07
3	New Hampshire	11.79
4	Alaska	11.08
5	Rhode Island	10.86
6	Maine	10.56
7	Massachusetts	10.53
8	New Mexico	10.35
9	Hawaii	10.23
10	Colorado	9.82
11	Nevada	9.58
12	South Dakota	9.57
13	Delaware	9.41
14	Oregon	9.31
15	Michigan	9.23
16	Connecticut	9.22
17	Nebraska	9.13
18	Washington	9.11
19	Minnesota	8.92
20	New York	8.76
21	Ohio	8.74
22	West Virginia	8.62
23	Florida	8.52
24	North Carolina	8.44
25	Virginia	8.43
26	Pennsylvania	8.18
27	Kentucky	8.16
28	Oklahoma	8.13
	National	8.03

Tables 2. States Ranked by Percentage of Youth Age 12-17 Reporting Past-Month Marijuana Use, 2002-2003 (Contiued)

Rank	State	%
29	*Arkansas*	7.97
30	Idaho	7.92
31	Maryland	7.87
32	Arizona	7.74
33	Wisconsin	7.71
34	California	7.66
35	Illinois	7.61
36	North Dakota	7.58
37	Missouri	7.43
	District of Columbia	7.43
38	Kansas	7.39
39	Indiana	7.37
40	New Jersey	7.33
41	South Carolina	7.25
42	Wyoming	7.14
43	Iowa	7.10
44	Louisiana	6.92
45	Georgia	6.87
46	Texas	6.38
47	Alabama	6.37
47	Tennessee	6.37
49	Mississippi	6.04
50	Utah	5.30

Source: SAMHSA, Office of Applied Studies, National Survey on Drug Use and Health, 2002 and 2003, Table B.3, at [http://www.oas. samhsa.gov/2k3State/appB.htm#tab B.3]. Rankings calculated by CRS.

The IOM Report further states (p. 126):

> Even if there were evidence that the medical use of marijuana would decrease the perception that it can be a harmful substance, this is beyond the scope of laws regulating the approval of therapeutic drugs. Those laws concern scientific data related to the safety and efficacy of drugs for individual use; they do not address perceptions or beliefs of the general population.

Tables 3. States Ranked by Percentage of Persons 12 or Older Reporting Past-Month Marijuana Use, 1999

Rank	State	%
1	Maryland	7.9
2	Colorado	7.7
3	Massachusetts	7.5
4	Rhode Island	7.4
5	Alaska	7.1
	District of Columbia	7.1
6	Washington	6.8
7	Oregon	6.6
8	Delaware	6.5
8	New Mexico	6.5
10	California	6.0
11	Montana	5.9
11	New Hampshire	5.9
13	Hawaii	5.8
13	Maine	5.8
15	Nevada	5.6
15	Wyoming	5.6
17	Vermont	5.4
18	Michigan	5.3
18	Minnesota	5.3
20	Arizona	5.2
21	Wisconsin	5.1
22	Connecticut	5.0
22	Florida	5.0
22	New Jersey	5.0
25	New York	4.9
25	Utah	4.9
	National	4.9
27	Illinois	4.8
29	Missouri	4.7
29	North Carolina	4.7
30	Indiana	4.6
31	Pennsylvania	4.5
32	Ohio	4.3
34	Georgia	4.2
34	Idaho	4.2
35	South Dakota	4.1
36	Virginia	4.0
38	Nebraska	3.9

Rank	State	%
38	North Dakota	3.9
39	South Carolina	3.8
40	Kansas	3.7
43	Kentucky	3.6
43	Tennessee	3.6
43	West Virginia	3.6
47	Arkansas	3.5
47	Louisiana	3.5
47	Oklahoma	3.5
47	Texas	3.5
50	Alabama	3.3
50	Iowa	3.3
50	Mississippi	3.3

Source: SAMHSA, Office of Applied Studies, National Household Survey on Drug Abuse, 1999, Table 3B, at [http://www.oas.samhsa.gov/NHSDA/99StateTabs/tables2.htm]. Rankings calculated by CRS.

Tables 4. States Ranked by Percentage of Persons 12 or Older Reporting Past-Month Marijuana Use, 2003-2004

Rank	State	%
1	New Hampshire	10.23
2	Alaska	9.78
3	Vermont	9.77
	District of Columbia	9.60
4	Rhode Island	9.56
5	Montana	9.17
6	Oregon	8.88
7	Colorado	8.49
8	Maine	7.95
9	Massachusetts	7.80
10	Nevada	7.62
11	Washington	7.41
12	New Mexico	7.37
13	New York	7.34
14	Michigan	7.20
15	Hawaii	6.95
16	Connecticut	9.94
17	Delaware	6.89
18	Missouri	6.76
19	Florida	6.58
20	California	6.50
21	Ohio	6.49

**Tables 4. States Ranked by Percentage of Persons 12 or Older Reporting
Past-Month Marijuana Use, 2003-2004 (Continued)**

22	Minnesota	6.37
	National	6.18
23	Indiana	6.12
24	Nebraska	5.97
25	Virginia	5.96
26	North Carolina	5.89
27	Louisiana	5.77
28	Maryland	5.73
29	Arizona	5.68
30	South Carolina	5.65
31	Pennsylvania	5.64
32	Arkansas	5.63
33	Kentucky	5.62
34	Illinois	5.60
35	Oklahoma	5.58
36	Wyoming	5.45
37	Wisconsin	5.40
38	North Dakota	5.35
39	South Dakota	5.24
40	West Virginia	5.12
41	Idaho	5.09
42	New Jersey	5.05
43	Georgia	4.93
44	Kansas	4.91
45	Iowa	4.90
46	Texas	4.79
47	Mississippi	4.64
48	Tennessee	4.59
49	Alabama	4.32
50	Utah	4.00

Source: SAMHSA, Office of Applied Studies, National Survey on Drug Use and Health,
2002 and 2003, Table B.3, at [http://www.oas.samhsa.gov/2k3State/appB.htm#
tabB.3]. Rankings calculated by CRS.

The IOM Report also found (p. 102): "No evidence suggests that the use of
opiates or cocaine for medical purposes has increased the perception that their
illicit use is safe or acceptable." Doctors can prescribe cocaine, morphine,
amphetamine, and methamphetamine, but this is not seen as weakening the War
on Drugs. Why would doctors recommending medical marijuana to their patients
be any different?

The so-called "Gateway Theory" of marijuana use is also cited to explain how medical marijuana could increase illicit drug use. With respect to the rationale behind the argument that marijuana serves as a "gateway" drug, the IOM Report offered the following (p. 6):

> In the sense that marijuana use typically precedes rather than follows initiation of other illicit drug use, it is indeed a "gateway" drug. But because underage smoking and alcohol use typically precede marijuana use, marijuana is not the most common, and is rarely the first, "gateway" to illicit drug use. There is no conclusive evidence that the drug effects of marijuana are causally linked to the subsequent abuse of other illicit drugs.

A statistical analysis of marijuana use by emergency room patients and arrestees in four states with medical marijuana programs — California, Colorado, Oregon, and Washington — found no statistically significant increase in recreational marijuana use among these two population subgroups after medical marijuana was approved for use. [111] Another study looked at adolescent marijuana use and found decreases in youth usage in every state with a medical marijuana law. Declines exceeding 50% were found in some age groups. [112]

These studies are consistent with the findings of a 2002 report by the Government Accountability Office that concluded that state medical marijuana laws were operating as voters and legislators intended and did not encourage drug use among the wider population. [113] Concerns that medical cannabis laws send the wrong message to vulnerable groups such as adolescents seem to be unfounded.

Medical Marijuana Undermines the War on Drugs

> The DEA and its local and state counterparts routinely report that large-scale drug traffickers hide behind and invoke Proposition 215, even when there is no evidence of any medical claim. In fact, many large-scale marijuana cultivators and traffickers escape state prosecution because of bogus medical marijuana claims. Prosecutors are reluctant to charge these individuals because of the state of confusion that exists in California. Therefore, high-level traffickers posing as 'care-givers' are able to sell illegal drugs with impunity.
> — "California Medical Marijuana Information," DEA Web page [114]

It is argued by many that state medical marijuana laws weaken the fight against drug abuse by making the work of police officers more difficult. This undermining of law enforcement can occur in at least three ways: by diverting medical marijuana into the recreational drug market, by causing state and local law enforcement priorities to diverge from federal priorities, and by complicating the job of law enforcement by forcing officers to distinguish medical users from recreational users.

Diversion. Marijuana grown for medical purposes, according to DEA and other federal drug control agencies, can be diverted into the larger, illegal marijuana market, thereby undermining law enforcement efforts to eliminate the marijuana market altogether. This point was emphasized by the Department of Justice (DOJ) in its prepublication review of a report by the Government Accountability Office (GAO) on medical marijuana. DOJ criticized the GAO draft report on the grounds that the "report did not mention that state medical marijuana laws are routinely abused to facilitate traditional illegal trafficking." [115]

GAO responded that in their interviews with federal officials regarding the impact of state medical marijuana laws on their law enforcement efforts, "none of the federal officials we spoke with provided information that abuse of medical marijuana laws was routinely occurring in any of the states, including California." [116] The government also failed to establish this in the Raich case. (It is of course possible that significant diversion is taking place yet remains undetected.)

Just as with many pharmaceuticals, some diversion is inevitable. Some would view this as an acceptable cost of implementing a medical marijuana program. Every public policy has its costs and benefits. Depriving seriously ill patients of their medical marijuana is seen by some as a small price to pay if doing so will help to protect America's youth from marijuana. Others balance the harms and benefits of medical marijuana in the opposite direction. Legal analyst Stuart Taylor Jr. recently wrote, "As a matter of policy, Congress as well as the states should legalize medical marijuana, with strict regulatory controls. The proven benefits to some suffering patients outweigh the potential costs of marijuana being diverted to illicit uses." [117]

Changed State and Local Law Enforcement Priorities. Following the passage of the California and Arizona medical marijuana initiatives in 1996, federal officials expressed concern that the measures would seriously affect the federal government's drug enforcement effort because federal drug policies rely heavily on the state's enforcement of their own drug laws to achieve federal objectives. For instance, in hearings before the Senate Judiciary Committee, the head of the Drug Enforcement Administration stated:

> I have always felt ... that the federalization of crime is very difficult to carry out; that crime, just in essence, is for the most part a local problem and addressed very well locally, in my experience. We now have a situation where local law enforcement is unsure.... The numbers of investigations that you would talk about that might be presently being conducted by the [Arizona state police] at the gram level would be beyond our capacity to conduct those types of individual investigations without abandoning the major organized crime investigations. [118]

State medical marijuana laws arguably feed into the deprioritization movement, by which drug reform advocates seek to influence state and local law enforcement to give a low priority to the enforcement of marijuana laws. This movement to make simple marijuana possession the lowest law enforcement priority has made inroads in such cities as San Francisco, Seattle, and Oakland, but it extends beyond the medical marijuana states to college towns such as Ann Arbor, MI, Madison, WI, Columbia, MO, and Lawrence, KS. [119] Federal officials fear that jurisdictions that "opt out" of marijuana enforcement "will quickly become a haven for drug traffickers." [120]

Distinguishing Between Legal and Illegal Providers and Users. Police officers in medical marijuana states have complained about the difficulty of distinguishing between legitimate patients and recreational marijuana smokers. According to the DEA:

> Local and state law enforcement counterparts cannot distinguish between illegal marijuana grows and grows that qualify as medical exemptions. Many self-designated medical marijuana growers are, in fact, growing marijuana for illegal, "recreational" use. [121]

This reasoning is echoed in the Raich amici brief of Community Rights Counsel (p. 12):

> Creating an exception for medical use [of marijuana] could undermine enforcement efforts by imposing an often difficult burden on prosecutors of establishing the violator's subjective motivation and intent beyond a reasonable doubt. Given that marijuana used in response to medical ailments is not readily distinguishable from marijuana used for other reasons, Congress rationally concluded that the control of all use is necessary to address the national market for controlled substances.

Patients and caregivers, on the other hand, have complained that their marijuana that is lawful under state statute has been seized by police and not returned. In some cases, patients and caregivers have been unexpectedly arrested by state or local police officers. A November 2002 GAO report on medical marijuana stated that "Several law enforcement officials in California and Oregon cited the inconsistency between federal and state law as a significant problem, particularly regarding how seized marijuana is handled." [122]

The failure of state and local law enforcement officers to observe state medical marijuana laws has especially been a problem in California. The California Highway Patrol (CHP) has, on numerous occasions, arrested patients or confiscated their medical marijuana during routine traffic stops. "Although voters legalized medical marijuana in California nearly nine years ago," reports the Los Angeles Times, "police statewide have wrangled with activists over how to enforce the law." [123]

As a result of a lawsuit brought against the CHP by a patient advocacy group, CHP officers will no longer seize patients' marijuana as long as they possess no more than 8 ounces and can show a certified-user identification card or their physician's written recommendation. The CHP's new policy, announced in August 2005, will likely influence the behavior of other California law enforcement agencies.

The Committee on Drugs and the Law of the Bar of the City of New York concluded its 1997 report "Marijuana Should be Medically Available" with this statement: "The government can effectively differentiate medical marijuana and recreational marijuana, as it has done with cocaine. The image of the Federal authorities suppressing a valuable medicine to maintain the rationale of the war on drugs only serves to discredit the government's effort." [124]

Patients Should Not Be Arrested for Using Medical Marijuana

> Centuries of Anglo-American law stand against the imposition of criminal liability on individuals for pursuing their own lifesaving pain relief and treatment.... Because the experience of pain can be so subversive of dignity — and even of the will to live — ethics and legal tradition recognize that individuals pursuing pain relief have special claims to non-interference.
> — Brief of the Leukemia and Lymphoma Society, et al., 2004 [125]

Medical marijuana advocates believe that seriously ill people should not be punished for acting in accordance with the opinion of their physicians in a bona fide attempt to relieve their suffering, especially when acting in accordance with state law. Even if marijuana were proven to be more harmful than now appears, prison for severely ill patients is believed to be a worse alternative. Patients have enough problems without having to fear the emotional and financial cost of arrest, legal fees, prosecution, and a possible prison sentence.

The American public appears to agree. The Institute of Medicine found that "public support for patient access to marijuana for medical use appears substantial; public opinion polls taken during 1997 and 1998 generally reported 60-70 percent of respondents in favor of allowing medical uses of marijuana." [126]

The federal penalty for possessing one marijuana cigarette — even for medical use — is up to one year in prison and up to a $100,000 fine, [127] and the penalty for growing a cannabis plant is up to five years and up to a $250,000 fine. [128] That patients are willing to risk these severe penalties to obtain the relief that marijuana provides appears to present strong evidence for the substance's therapeutic effectiveness.

Although the Supreme Court ruled differently in Raich, the argument persists that medical marijuana providers and patients are engaging in a class of activity totally different from those persons trafficking in marijuana for recreational use and that patients should not be arrested for using medical marijuana in accordance with the laws of the states in which they reside.

With its position affirmed by Raich, however, DEA continues to investigate — and sometimes raid and shut down — medical marijuana distribution operations in California and other medical marijuana states. DEA's position is that:

> [F]ederal law does not distinguish between crimes involving marijuana for claimed "medical" purposes and crimes involving marijuana for any other purpose. DEA likewise does not so distinguish in carrying out its duty to enforce the CSA and investigate possible violations of the Act. Rather, consistent with the agency's mandate, DEA focuses on large-scale trafficking organizations and other criminal enterprises that warrant federal scrutiny. If investigating CSA violations in this manner leads the agency to encounter persons engaged in criminal activities involving marijuana, DEA does not alter its approach if such persons claim at some point their crimes are "medically" justified. To do so would be to give legal effect to an excuse considered by the text of federal law and the United States Supreme Court to be of no moment. [129]

Because nearly all arrests and prosecutions for marijuana possession are handled by state and local law enforcement officers, patients and caregivers in the medical marijuana states can, as a practical matter, possess medical marijuana without fear of arrest and imprisonment. DEA enforcement actions against medical marijuana dispensaries — as occurred in San Francisco shortly after the Raich decision was announced [130] — can, however, make it more difficult for patients to obtain the drug. The situation that Grinspoon and Bakalar described in 1995 in the Journal of the American Medical Association persists a decade later: "At present, the greatest danger in medical use of marihuana is its illegality, which imposes much anxiety and expense on suffering people, forces them to bargain with illicit drug dealers, and exposes them to the threat of criminal prosecution." [131]

The States Should Be Allowed to Experiment

> Doctors, not the federal government, know what's best for their patients. If a
> state decides to allow doctors to recommend proven treatments for their patients,
> then the federal government has no rightful place in the doctor's office.
> — Attorney Randy Barnett, 2004 [132]

Three States — California, Maryland, and Washington — filed an amici curiae brief supporting the right of states to institute medical marijuana programs. Their brief argued, "In our federal system States often serve as democracy's laboratories, trying out new, or innovative solutions to society's ills." [133]

The Raich case shows that the federal government has zero tolerance for state medical marijuana programs. The Bush Administration appealed the decision of the Ninth Circuit Court of Appeals to the Supreme Court, which reversed the Ninth Circuit and upheld the federal position against the states. Framed as a Commerce Clause issue, the case became a battle for states' rights against the federal government.

The Raich case created unusual political alliances. Three southern states that are strongly opposed to any marijuana use, medical or otherwise — Alabama, Louisiana, and Mississippi — filed an amici curiae brief supporting California's medical marijuana users on the grounds of states' rights. Their brief argued

> As Justice Brandeis famously remarked, "[i]t is one of the happy incidents
> of the federal system that a single courageous State may, if its citizens choose,
> serve as a laboratory; and try novel social and economic experiments without risk
> to the rest of the country." [134] Whether California and the other
> compassionate-use States are "courageous — or instead profoundly misguided —
> is not the point. The point is that, as a sovereign member of the federal union,
> California is entitled to make for itself the tough policy choices that affect its
> citizens. [135]

States' rights advocates argue that authority to define criminal law and the power to make and enforce laws protecting the health, safety, welfare, and morals reside at the state level and that a state has the right to set these policies free of congressional interference.

For Justice O'Connor, the Raich case exemplified "the role of States as laboratories." [136] She wrote in her dissenting opinion:

> If I were a California citizen, I would not have voted for the medical marijuana ballot initiative; if I were a California legislator I would not have supported the Compassionate Use Act. But whatever the wisdom of California's experiment with medical marijuana, the federalism principles that have driven our Commerce Clause cases require that room for experiment be protected in this case. [137]

Medical Marijuana Laws Harm the Drug Approval Process

> The current efforts to gain legal status of marijuana through ballot initiatives seriously threaten the Food and Drug Administration statutorily authorized process of proving safety and efficacy.
>   — Brief of the Drug Free America Foundation, et al., 2004 [138]

Although the individual states regulate the practice of medicine, the federal government has taken primary responsibility for the regulation of medical products, especially those containing controlled substances. Pharmaceutical drugs must be approved for use in the United States by the Food and Drug Administration, an agency of the Department of Health and Human Services. The Federal Food, Drug, and Cosmetics Act gives HHS and FDA the responsibility for determining that drugs are safe and effective, a requirement that all medicines must meet before they can enter interstate commerce and be made available for general medical use. [139] Clinical evaluation is required regardless of whether the drug is synthetically produced or originates from a natural botanical or animal source.

Opponents of medical marijuana say that the FDA's drug approval process should not be circumvented. To permit states to decide which medical products can be made available for therapeutic use, they say, would undercut this regulatory system. State medical marijuana initiatives are seen as inconsistent with the federal government's responsibility to protect the public from unsafe, ineffective drugs.

The Bush Administration argued in its brief in the Raich case that "excepting drug activity for personal use or free distribution from the sweep of [federal drug laws] would discourage the consumption of lawful controlled substances and would undermine Congress's intent to regulate the drug market comprehensively to protect public health and safety." [140]

Three prominent drug abuse experts argued in their amici brief:

> This action by the state of California did not create a "novel social and economic experiment," but rather chaos in the scientific and medical communities. Furthermore, under Court of Appeals ruling, such informal State systems could be replicated, and even expanded, in a manner that puts at risk the critical protections so carefully crafted under the national food and drug legislation of the 20th century. [141]

The Food and Drug Administration itself has stated that

> FDA is the sole Federal agency that approves drug products as safe and effective for intended indications.... FDA's drug approval process requires well-controlled clinical trials that provide the necessary scientific data upon which FDA makes its approval and labeling decisions.... Efforts that seek to bypass the FDA drug approval process would not serve the interests of public health because they might expose patients to unsafe and ineffective drug products. FDA has not approved smoked marijuana for any condition or disease indication. [142]

The Drug Free America Raich brief elaborates further (pp. 12-13):

> The ballot initiative-led laws create an atmosphere of medicine by popular vote, rather than the rigorous scientific and medical process that all medicines must undergo. Before the development of modern pharmaceutical science, the field of medicine was fraught with potions and herbal remedies. Many of those were absolutely useless, or conversely were harmful to unsuspecting subjects. Thus evolved our current Food and Drug Administration and drug scheduling processes, which Congress has authorized in order to create a uniform and reliable system of drug approval and regulation. This system is being intentionally undermined by the legalization proponents through use of medical marijuana initiatives.

The organizers of the medical marijuana state initiatives deny that it was their intent to undermine the federal drug approval process. Rather, in their view, it became necessary for them to bypass the FDA and go to the states because of the federal government's resistance to marijuana research requests and rescheduling petitions.

As for the charge that politics should not play a role in the drug approval and controlled substance scheduling processes, medical marijuana supporters point out that marijuana's original listing as a Schedule I substance in 1970 was itself a political act on the part of Congress.

Scientists on both sides of the issue say more research needs to be done, yet some researchers charge that the federal government has all but shut down marijuana clinical trials for reasons based on politics and ideology rather than science. [143]

In any case, as the IOM Report pointed out, "although a drug is normally approved for medical use only on proof of its 'safety and efficacy,' patients with life- threatening conditions are sometimes (under protocols for 'compassionate use') allowed access to unapproved drugs whose benefits and risks are uncertain." [144] This was the case with the FDA's IND Compassionate Access Program under which a limited number of patients are provided government-grown medical marijuana to treat their serious medical conditions.

Some observers believe the pharmaceutical industry and some politicians oppose medical marijuana to protect pharmaceutical industry profits. Because the whole marijuana plant cannot be patented, research efforts must be focused on the development of synthetic cannabinoids such as Marinol. But even if additional cannabinoid drugs are developed and marketed, some believe that doctors and patients should still not be criminalized for recommending and using the natural substance.

The New England Journal of Medicine has editorialized that

> [A] federal policy that prohibits physicians from alleviating suffering by prescribing marijuana for seriously ill patients is misguided, heavy-handed, and inhumane. Marijuana may have long-term adverse effects and its use may presage serious addictions, but neither long-term side effects nor addiction is a relevant issue in such patients. It is also hypocritical to forbid physicians to prescribe marijuana while permitting them to use morphine and meperidine to relieve extreme dyspnea and pain. With both of these drugs the difference between the dose that relieves symptoms and the dose that hastens death is very narrow; by contrast, there is no risk of death from smoking marijuana. To demand evidence of therapeutic efficacy is equally hypocritical. The noxious sensations that patients experience are extremely difficult to quantify in controlled experiments. What really counts for a therapy with this kind of safety margin is whether a seriously ill patient feels relief as a result of the intervention, not whether a controlled trial "proves" its efficacy. [145]

Some observers suggest that until the federal government relents and becomes more hospitable to marijuana research proposals and more willing to consider moving marijuana to a less restrictive schedule, the medical marijuana issue will continue to be fought at state and local levels of governance. As one patient advocate has stated, "As the months tick away, it will become more and more obvious that we need to continue changing state laws until the federal government has no choice but to change its inhumane medicinal marijuana laws." [146]

The Medical Marijuana Movement Is Politically Inspired

> Advocates have tried to legalize marijuana in one form or another for three decades, and the "medical marijuana" concept is a Trojan Horse tactic towards the goal of legalization.
> — Brief of the Drug Free America Foundation, et al., 2004 [147]

Medical marijuana opponents see the movement to promote the use of medical marijuana as a cynical attempt to subvert the Controlled Substances Act and legalize the recreational use of marijuana for all. They see it as a devious tactic in the more than 30-year effort by marijuana proponents to bring an end to marijuana prohibition in the United States and elsewhere.

They point out that between 1972 and 1978, the National Organization for the Reform of Marijuana Laws (NORML) successfully lobbied 11 state legislatures to decriminalize the drug, reducing penalties for possession in most cases to that of a traffic ticket. Also, in 1972, NORML began the first of several unsuccessful attempts to petition DEA to reschedule marijuana from Schedule I to Schedule II on the grounds that crude marijuana had use in medicine. [148]

Later, beginning with California in 1996, "drug legalizers" pushed successfully for passage of medical marijuana voter initiatives in several states, prompting then-Drug Czar Barry McCaffrey, writing in Newsweek, to warn that "We're on a Perilous Path." "I think it's clear," he wrote, "that a lot of the people arguing for the California proposition and others like it are pushing the legalization of drugs, plain and simple." [149]

Is it cynical or smart for NORML and other drug reform organizations to simultaneously pursue the separate goals of marijuana decriminalization for all, on the one hand, and marijuana rescheduling for the seriously ill, on the other? It is not unusual for political activists tactically to press for — and accept — half-measures in pursuit of a larger strategic goal. Pro-life activists work to prohibit partial-birth abortions and to pass parental notification laws. Gay rights activists seek limited domestic partner benefits as a stepping stone to full marriage equality. Thus is the tactic used on both sides of the cultural divide in America, to the alarm of those opposed.

It is certainly true that the medical cannabis movement is an offshoot of the marijuana legalization movement. Many individuals and organizations that support medical marijuana also support a broader program of drug law reform. It is also true, however, that many health professionals and other individuals who advocate medical access to marijuana do not support any other changes in U.S. drug control policy. In the same way, not everyone in favor of parental notification laws supports banning abortions for everyone. And not every supporter of domestic partner benefits believes in same-sex marriage.

In these hot-button issues, ideology and emotion often rule. Marijuana users in general, and medical marijuana users in particular, are demonized by some elements of American society. The ideology of the "Drug Warriors" intrudes on the science of medical marijuana, as pointed out by Grinspoon and Bakalar in the Journal of the American Medical Association:

> Advocates of medical use of marihuana are sometimes charged with using medicine as a wedge to open a way for "recreational" use. The accusation is false as applied to its target, but expresses in a distorted form a truth about some opponents of medical marihuana: they will not admit that it can be a safe and effective medicine largely because they are stubbornly committed to exaggerating its dangers when used for nonmedical purposes. [150]

The authors of the IOM Report were aware of the possibility that larger ideological positions could influence one's stand on the specific issue of patient access to medical marijuana when they wrote that

> [I]t is not relevant to scientific validity whether an argument is put forth by someone who believes that all marijuana use should be legal or by someone who believes that any marijuana use is highly damaging to individual users and to society as a whole. (p. 14)

In other words, it is widely believed that science should rule when it comes to medical issues. Both sides in the medical marijuana debate claim adherence to this principle. The House Government Reform Committee's April 2004 hearing on medical marijuana was titled "Marijuana and Medicine: The Need for a Science-Based Approach." And medical marijuana advocates plead with the federal government to permit scientific research on medical marijuana to proceed.

Rescheduling marijuana and making it available for medical use and research is not necessarily a step toward legalizing its recreational use. Such a move would put it on a par with cocaine, methamphetamine, morphine, and methadone, all of which are Schedule II substances that are not close to becoming legal for recreational use. Proponents of medical marijuana ask why marijuana should be considered differently than these other scheduled substances.

It is also arguable that marijuana should indeed be considered differently than cocaine, methamphetamine, morphine, and methadone. Scientists note that marijuana is less harmful and less addictive than these Schedule II substances. Acceptance of medical marijuana could in fact pave the way for its more generalized use. Ethan Nadelmann, head of the Drug Policy Alliance, has observed, "As medical marijuana becomes more regulated and institutionalized in the West, that may provide a model for how we ultimately make marijuana legal for all adults." [151] Medical marijuana opponents have trumpeted his candor as proof of the hypocrisy of those on the other side of the issue. Others note, however, that his comment may be less hypocritical than astute.

REFERENCE

[1]   The terms medical marijuana and medical cannabis are used interchangeably in this report to refer to marijuana (scientific name: Cannabis sativa) and to marijuana use that qualifies for a medical use exception under the laws of certain states and under the federal Investigational New Drug Compassionate Access Program.

[2]   The terms botanical cannabis, herbal cannabis, botanical marijuana, and crude marijuana, used interchangeably in this report, signify the whole or parts of the natural marijuana plant and therapeutic products derived therefrom, as opposed to drugs produced synthetically in the laboratory that replicate molecules found in the marijuana plant.

[3]   Gregg A. Bliz, "The Medical Use of Marijuana: The Politics of Medicine," *Hamline Journal of Public Law and Policy*, vol. 13, spring 1992, p. 118.

[4]   Oakley Ray and Charles Ksir, Drugs, Society, and Human Behavior, 10th ed. (New York: McGraw-Hill, 2004), p. 456.

[5]   Bill Zimmerman, Is Marijuana the Right Medicine for You? A Factual Guide to Medical Uses of Marijuana (New Canaan, CT: Keats Publishing, 1998), p. 19.

[6]   In Spanish, the letter "j" carries the sound of "h" in English. This alternative spelling of marijuana (with an "h") was formerly used by the federal government and is still used by some writers today.

[7]   P.L. 75-238, 50 Stat. 551, August 2, 1937. In Leary v. United States (395 U.S. 6 (1968)), the Supreme Court ruled the Marihuana Tax Act unconstitutional because it compelled self- incrimination, in violation of the Fifth Amendment.

[8]   P.L. 63-223, December 17, 1914, 38 Stat. 785. This law was passed to implement the Hague Convention of 1912 and created a federal tax on opium and coca leaves and their derivatives.

[9]   U.S. Congress, House Committee on Ways and Means, Taxation of Marihuana, hearings on H.R. 6385, 75th Cong., 1st sess., May 4, 1937 (Washington: GPO, 1937), p. 114.

[10] U.S. Congress, Senate Committee on Finance, Taxation of Marihuana, hearing on H.R. 6906, 75th Cong., 1st sess., July 12, 1937 (Washington: GPO, 1937), p. 33.

[11] U.S. President, 1969-1974 (Nixon), "Special Message to the Congress on Control of Narcotics and Dangerous Drugs," July 14, 1969, Public Papers of the Presidents of the United States 1969 (Washington: GPO, 1971), pp. 513-518.

[12] U.S. Congress, Conference Committees, Comprehensive Drug Abuse Prevention and Control Act of 1970, conference report to accompany H.R. 18583, 91st Cong., 2nd sess., H.Rept. 91-1603 (Washington: GPO, 1970).

[13] Title II of the Comprehensive Drug Abuse Prevention and Control Act of 1970, P.L. 91- 513, October 27, 1970, 84 Stat. 1242, 21 U.S.C. §801, et seq.

[14] Ibid., Sec. 202(b)(1), 84 Stat. 1247, 21 U.S.C. §812(b)(1).

[15] Ibid., Sec. 202(c), 84 Stat. 1248.

[16] Ibid., Sec. 404 (21 U.S.C. §844) and 18 U.S.C. §3571. Sec. 404 also calls for a minimum fine of $1,000, and Sec. 405 (21 U.S.C. §844a) permits a civil penalty of up to $10,000.

[17] Sec. 102(15), (22) of the CSA (21 U.S.C. §802(15), (22)).

[18] Sec. 401(b)(1)(D) of the CSA (21 U.S.C. §841(b)(1)(D)).

[19] Omnibus Consolidated and Emergency Supplemental Appropriations Act, 1999, P.L. 105- 277, October 21, 1998, 112 Stat. 2681-760.

[20] Ibid., District of Columbia Appropriations Act, 1999, Sec. 171, 112 Stat. 268 1-150.

[21] "The Legalization of Marijuana for Medical Treatment Initiative of 1998, also known as Initiative 59, approved by the electors of the District of Columbia on November 3, 1998, shall not take effect." (District of

Columbia Appropriations Act, 2006 (Division B of P.L. 109-115, Sec. 128 (b); 119 Stat. 2521.) This recurring provision of D.C. appropriations acts is known as the Barr Amendment because it was originally offered by Rep. Bob Barr. Since leaving Congress in 2003, Barr changed his position and is now working in support of medical marijuana as a lobbyist for the Marijuana Policy Project. See his website [http://www.bobbarr.org].

[22] When last considered in July 2007, the amendment stated: "None of the funds made available in this Act to the Department of Justice may be used, with respect to the States of Alaska, California, Colorado, Hawaii, Maine, Montana, Nevada, New Mexico, Oregon, Rhode Island, Vermont, and Washington, to prevent such States from implementing their own State laws that authorize the use, distribution, possession, or cultivation of medical marijuana." The wording of previous versions of the amendment was similar.

[23] "Amendment No. 1 offered by Mr. Hinchey," Congressional Record, daily edition, vol. 149 (July 22, 2003), pp. H7302-H73 11 and vol. 149 (July 23, 2003), pp. H7354-H7355.

[24] "Amendment No. 6 Offered by Mr. Farr," Congressional Record, daily edition, vol. 150 (July 7, 2004), pp. H5300-H5306, H5320.

[25] 25 "Amendment Offered by Mr. Hinchey," Congressional Record, daily edition, vol. 151 (July 15, 2005), pp. H4519-H4524, H4529.

[26] "Amendment Offered by Mr. Hinchey," Congressional Record, daily edition, vol. 152 (June 28, 2006), pp. H4735-H4739.

[27] 27 "Amendment Offered by Mr. Hinchey," Congressional Record, daily edition, vol. 153 (July 25, 2007), p. H8484.

[28] For a legal analysis of the amendment, see CRS Congressional Distribution Memorandum, "Possible Legal Effects of the Medical Marijuana Amendment to S. 1082," by Vanessa Burrows and Brian Yeh.

[29] "Frank Introduces Legislation to Remove Federal Penalties on Personal Marijuana Use," press release from the office of Rep. Barney Frank, April 17, 2008.

[30] The Common Law Doctrine of Necessity argues that the illegal act committed (in this case, growing marijuana) was necessary to avert a greater harm (blindness).

[31] Despite the program's name, it was not a clinical trial to test the drug for eventual approval, but a means for the government to provide medical marijuana to patients demonstrating necessity. Some have criticized the government for its failure to study the safety and efficacy of the medical-grade marijuana it grew and distributed to this patient population.

[32] U.S. Dept. of Justice, Drug Enforcement Administration, "Schedules of Controlled Substances: Rescheduling of Synthetic Dronobinol in Sesame Oil and Encapsulation in Soft Gelatin Capsules From Schedule I to Schedule II; Statement of Policy," 51 *Federal Register* 17476, May 13, 1986.

[33] Ibid., "Schedules of Controlled Substances: Rescheduling of the Food and Drug Administration Approved Product Containing Synthetic Dronabinol [(-)-delta nine-(trans)- Tetrahydrocannabinol] in Sesame Oil and Encapsulated in Soft Gelatin Capsules From Schedule II to Schedule III," 64 *Federal Register* 35928, July 2, 1999.

[34] Ibid., Bureau of Narcotics and Dangerous Drugs, "Schedule of Controlled Substances: Petition to Remove Marijuana or in the Alternative to Control Marijuana in Schedule V of the Controlled Substances Act," 37 *Federal Register* 18097, September 7, 1972.

[35] Ibid., Drug Enforcement Administration, "In the Matter of Marijuana Rescheduling Petition, Docket No. 86-22, Opinion and Recommended Ruling, Findings of Fact, Conclusions of Law and Decision of Administrative Law Judge," Francis L. Young, Administrative Law Judge, September 6, 1988. This quote and the following two quotes are at pp. 58-59, 68, and 67, respectively. This opinion is online at [http://www.druglibrary.net/ olsen/MEDICAL/YOUNG/young.html].

[36] Ibid., "Marijuana Scheduling Petition; Denial of Petition," 54 Federal Register 53767 at 53768, December 29, 1989. The petition denial was appealed, eventually resulting in yet another DEA denial to reschedule. See Ibid., "Marijuana Scheduling Petition; Denial of Petition; Remand," 57 *Federal Register* 10499, March 26, 1992.

[37] National Institutes of Health. The Ad Hoc Group of Experts. Workshop on the Medical Utility of Marijuana: Report to the Director, August 1997. (Hereafter cited as NIH Workshop.) [http://www.nih.gov/news/ medmarijuana/MedicalMarijuana.htm]

[38] Janet E. Joy, Stanley J. Watson, Jr., and John A. Benson, Jr., eds., Marijuana and Medicine: Assessing the Science Base (Washington: National Academy Press, 1999). (Hereafter cited as the IOM Report.) [http://www.nap.edu/books/030907 1550/html/]

[39] U.S. Dept. of Justice, Drug Enforcement Administration, "Notice of Denial of Petition," 65 *Federal Register* 20038, April 18, 2001.

[40] U.S. Food and Drug Administration, "Inter-Agency Advisory Regarding Claims That Smoked Marijuana Is a Medicine," press release, April 20, 2006, p. 1. Although not cited in the press release, the "past evaluation"

referred to is apparently the 2001 denial of the petition to reschedule marijuana discussed above.

[41] See, for example, "The Politics of Pot," editorial, New York Times, April 22, 2006, p. A26, which calls the FDA statement "disingenuous" and concludes: "It's obviously easier and safer to issue a brief, dismissive statement than to back research that might undermine the administration's inflexible opposition to the medical use of marijuana."

[42] The text of the letter, dated April 27, 2006, is available at Rep. Hinchey's website [http://www.house.gov/hinchey].

[43] Jessica Winter, "Weed Control: Research on the Medicinal Benefits of Marijuana May Depend on Good Gardening — and Some Say Uncle Sam, the Country's Only Legal Grower of the Cannabis Plant, Isn't Much of a Green Thumb," Boston Globe, May 28, 2006.

[44] "The UMass Amherst MMJ Production Facility Project," on the MAPS website at [http://www.maps.org/mmj/mmjfacility.html]. See the entry for February 8, 2005. (Numerous documents related to the Craker/MAPS application are linked here.)

[45] U.S. Dept. of Justice, Drug Enforcement Administration, "In the Matter Lyle E. Craker, Ph.D., Docket No. 05-16, Opinion and Recommended Ruling, Findings of Fact, Conclusions of Law, and Decision of Administrative Law Judge," Mary Ellen Bittner, Administrative Law Judge, February 12, 2007, p. 87. This opinion is online at [ttp://www.maps.org/ mmj/ DEAlawsuit.html].

[46] Rone Tempest, "DEA Targets Larger Marijuana Providers," Los Angeles Times, January 1, 2007.

[47] These include medical marijuana activist and author Ed Rosenthal, whose first jury renounced its guilty verdict when it learned after the trial that he was legally helping patients under state law and who is being tried again. See Paul Elias, "Federal Prosecutors Will Retry Ed Rosenthal Against Judge Recommendation," Associated Press, April 15, 2007.

[48] Sec. 416 of the Controlled Substances Act (21 U.S.C. § 856) as amended by P.L. 99-570, Title I, sec. 1841(a), October 27, 1986; 100 Stat. 3207-52. Actually, the crack house statute was amended in 2003 by the "rave act" (§ 608 of P.L. 108-21, May 1, 2003; 117 Stat. 691), which broadened the language of the crack house statute to include outdoor venues and other possible places where raves could be held by striking the words "building, room, or enclosure" (which appear in the DEA letter) and replacing them with "place." This and other subtle but significant changes in the language of the law were designed to penalize rave promoters and the owners and

managers of the venues where raves (all-night music festivals) occur at which Ecstasy (MDMA) and other club drugs might be used. The July 2007 DEA letter cites the language of the pre-2003 version of the crack house statute rather than the provision of law currently in force. This section of the CSA has also been used by the DEA against fund-raising events put on by drug law reform organizations.

[49] 21 U.S.C. § 881(a)(7).
[50] "New Challenges for Medical Marijuana," Los Angeles Times editorial, July 19, 2007.
[51] County of Santa Cruz v. Ashcroft, 314 F.Supp.2d 1000 (N.D.Cal. 2004); the decision, however, rests on the 9th Circuit's ruling in Raich, subsequently reversed by the Supreme Court, as described below.
[52] For a legal analysis of the three Supreme Court cases mentioned here, see CRS Report RL3 1100, Marijuana for Medical Purposes: The Supreme Court's Decision in United States v. Oakland Cannabis Buyers' Cooperative and Related Legal Issues, by Charles Doyle.
[53] The necessity defense argues that the illegal act committed (distribution of marijuana in this instance) was necessary to avert a greater harm (withholding a helpful drug from seriously ill patients).
[54] 190 F.3d 1109.
[55] 532 U.S. 483 (2001) at 494 n. 7.
[56] Conant v. McCaffrey, 172 F.R.D. 681 (N.D. Cal. 1997).
[57] Conant v. Walters, 309 F.3d 629, 636 (9th Cir. 2002); the parties agreed that "a doctor who actually prescribes or dispenses marijuana violates federal law," ibid. at 634.
[58] Raich v. Ashcroft, 352 F.3d 1222 (9th Cir. 2003).
[59] Gonzales v. Raich, 125 S.Ct. 2195, 2205 (2005).
[60] Ibid. at 2211 n. 37. For a legal analysis of this case, see CRS Report RS22 167, Gonzales v. Raich: Congress's Power Under the Commerce Clause to Regulate Medical Marijuana, by Todd B. Tatelman.
[61] Ibid. at 2215.
[62] P.L. 106-554, 114 Stat. 2763A-153, 44 U.S.C. § 3516 note. For background on the DQA see CRS Report RL32532, The Information Quality Act: OMB's Guidance and Initial Implementation, by Curtis W. Copeland.
[63] The original petition and all subsequent documents relating to the case can be found at [http://www.safeaccessnow.org/article.php?id=440 1]. See also Carolyn Marshall, "U.S. Is Sued Over Position on Marijuana," New York Times, February 22, 2007.

[64] The information in this and the following section is drawn largely from: State-by-State Medical Marijuana Laws: How to Remove the Threat of Arrest, Marijuana Policy Project, July 2004, available at [http://www.mpp. org/statelaw/index.html]. More recent information is from press reports.

[65] Alaska (Stat. § 11.71.090); California (Cal.Health and Safety Code Ann. § 11362.5) and (2003 CA S.B. 420 (SN)); Colorado (Colo.Const. Art. XVIII § 14); Hawaii (Rev.Stat. §§329-121 to 329-128); Maine (Me.Rev.Stat.Ann. tit.22 §1102 or 2382-B(5)); Montana (Mont.Code Ann. §§50-46-101 to 50-46-210); Nevada (Nev.Rev.Stat.Ann. §§453A.010 to 453A.400); New Mexico (S.B. 523); Oregon (Ore.Rev.Stat. §§475.300 to 475.346); Rhode Island (RI ST §§21-28.6-1); Vermont (Vt.Stat.Ann. tit. 18, §§4472-4474d); Washington (Wash.Rev.Code Ann. § 69.5 1A.005 to 69.5 1A.902).

[66] Dale Gieringer, "The Acceptance of Medical Marijuana in the U.S.," *Journal of Cannabis Therapeutics*, vol. 3, no. 1 (2003), pp. 53-67. The author later estimated that there were more than 100,000 medical marijuana patients in California alone (personal communication dated April 30, 2004).

[67] Susan Okie, "Medical Marijuana and the Supreme Court," *New England Journal of Medicine,* vol. 353, no. 7 (August 18, 2005), p. 649.

[68] The telephone survey was conducted for this report by CRS summer intern Broocks Andrew Meade.

[69] Ariz.Rev.Stat.Ann. §13-3412.01(A).

[70] Md. Crim.Code Ann. §5-601.

[71] State-by-State Medical Marijuana Laws: How to Remove the Threat of Arrest, Marijuana Policy Project, July 2004, p. 3. The laws in some of these states have expired or been repealed.

[72] For more information on the situation in the District of Columbia, see CRS Report RL33563, District of Columbia: Appropriations for 2007, by Eugene Boyd and David P. Smole.

[73] The questions asked and the results obtained can be viewed at [http://www.medicalmarijuanaprocon.org/pop/votesNat.htm].

[74] Robert J. Blend on and John T. Young, "The Public and the War on Illicit Drugs," *Journal of the American Medical Association*, vol. 279, no. 11 (March 18, 1998), p. 831.

[75] Brief for the Drug Free America Foundation, Inc. et al. as Amici Curiae Supporting Petitioners at 13, Gonzales v. Raich, 125 S.Ct. 2195 (2005) (No. 03-1454). The amici curiae briefs filed in Raich contain a wealth of information and arguments on both sides of the medical marijuana debate. They are available online at [http://www.angeljustice.org].

[76] See, for example, "Exposing the Myth of Medical Marijuana," on the DEA website at [http://www.usdoj .gov/dea/ongoing/marijuanap.html].

[77] Ibid., at 25.

[78] This test was first formulated by the DEA in 1992 in response to a marijuana rescheduling petition. See U.S. Department of Justice, Drug Enforcement Administration, "Marijuana Scheduling Petition; Denial of Petition; Remand," 57 *Federal Register* 10499, March 26, 1992, at 10506.

[79] Ibid., p. 10507.

[80] Ibid., pp. 10506-10507.

[81] Gonzales v. Raich, 125 S.Ct. 2195, at 2212 and 2213 (2005).

[82] Brief for the Leukemia and Lymphoma Society, et al. as Amici Curiae Supporting Respondents at 4, Gonzales v. Raich, 125 S.Ct. 2195 (2005) (No. 03-1454).

[83] Ibid., at 1-2.

[84] A 1990 survey of oncologists found that 54% of those with an opinion on medical marijuana favored the controlled medical availability of marijuana and 44% had already broken the law by suggesting at least once that a patient obtain marijuana illegally. R. Doblin and M. Kleiman, "Marijuana as Antiemetic Medicine," *Journal of Clinical Oncology*, vol. 9 (1991), pp. 1314-1319.

[85] There is evidence that marijuana might also be useful in treating arthritis, migraine, menstrual cramps, alcohol and opiate addiction, and depression and other mood disorders.

[86] IOM Report, pp. 3-4: "The effects of cannabinoids on the symptoms studied are generally modest, and in most cases there are more effective medications. However, people vary in their responses to medications, and there will likely always be a subpopulation of patients who do not respond well to other medications."

[87] Brief for the Leukemia and Lymphoma Society et al. as Amici Curiae Supporting Respondents at 18, Gonzales v. Raich, 125 S.Ct. 2195 (2005) (No. 03-1454).

[88] Marinol currently sells at retail for about $17 per pill.

[89] "Federal Foolishness and Marijuana," *New England Journal of Medicine,* vol. 336, no. 5 (January 30, 1997), pp. 366-367.

[90] The website "Medical Marijuana ProCon" [http://www.medicalmarijuana-procon.org] contains information on organizations that both support and oppose medical marijuana.

[91] For a summary of the growing body of research on endocannabinoids, see Roger A. Nicoll and Bradley N. Alger, "The Brain's Own Marijuana,"

Scientific American, December 2004, pp. 68-75, and Jean Marx, "Drugs Inspired by a Drug," *Science,* January 20, 2006, pp. 322- 325.

[92] Bill Zimmerman, Is Marijuana the Right Medicine For You? A Factual Guide to Medical Uses of Marijuana (Keats Publishing, New Canaan, CT: 1998), p. 25.

[93] Barry R. McCaffrey, "We're on a Perilous Path," Newsweek, February 3, 1997, p. 27.

[94] Karen Tandy, "Marijuana: The Myths Are Killing Us," Police Chief Magazine, March 2005, available at [http://www.usdoj.gov/dea/pubs/ pressrel/pr042605p.html].

[95] Lynn Zimmer and John P. Morgan, Marijuana Myths Marijuana Facts (New York: Lindesmith Center, 1997), p. 115.

[96] Medicines do not have to be completely safe to be approved. In fact, no medicine is completely safe; every drug has toxicity concerns. All pharmaceuticals have potentially harmful side effects, and it would be startling, indeed, if botanical marijuana were found to be an exception. The IOM Report states that "except for the harms associated with smoking, the adverse effects of marijuana use are within the range of effects tolerated for other medications." (p. 5)

[97] American Medical Association, Council on Scientific Affairs Report: Medical Marijuana (A-01), June 2001. An unpaginated version of this document can be found on the Web at [http://www.mfiles.org/Marijuana/ medicinal_use/b2_ama_csa_report.html].

[98] Cannabis preparations are also used topically as oils and balms to soothe muscles, tendons, and joints.

[99] Several companies offer vaporizers for sale in the United States, but their marketing is complicated by marijuana prohibition and by laws prohibiting drug paraphernalia. The advantages of the vaporizer were brought to the attention of the IOM panel. The IOM Report, however, devoted only one sentence to such devices, despite its recommendation for research into safe delivery systems. The IOM Report said, "Vaporization devices that permit inhalation of plant cannabinoids without the carcinogenic combustion products found in smoke are under development by several groups; such devices would also require regulatory review by the FDA." (p. 216)

[100] U.S. Dept. of Justice, Drug Enforcement Administration, "In the Matter of Marijuana Rescheduling Petition, Docket No. 86-22, Opinion and Recommended Ruling, Findings of Fact, Conclusions of Law and Decision of Administrative Law Judge," Francis L. Young, Administrative Law

Judge, September 6, 1988, p. 67. This opinion is online at [http://www.druglibrary.net/olsen/MEDICAL/YOUNG/young.html].

[101] Ibid., pp. 58-59.

[102] Ibid., p. 56.

[103] When Congress directly schedules a drug, as it did marijuana in 1970, it is not bound by the criteria in section 202(b) of the CSA (21 U.S.C. 812(b)).

[104] Congress could also follow the lead of some states that have a dual scheduling scheme for botanical marijuana whereby its recreational use is prohibited (Schedule I) but it is permitted when used for medicinal purposes (Schedules II or III). Congress could achieve the same effect by leaving marijuana in Schedule I but removing criminal penalties for the medical use of marijuana, commonly called decriminalization. Congress could also opt for legalization by removing marijuana from the CSA entirely and subjecting it to federal and state controls based on the tobacco or alcohol regulatory models or by devising a regulatory scheme unique to marijuana. None of these options seem likely given the current political climate in which both political parties support marijuana prohibition.

[105] These and other poll results can be consulted at [http://www.medical-marijuanaprocon.org/ pop/votes.htm]. This website states: "Because 100% of the voter initiatives and polls we located were favorable (50.01% or more pro) towards the medical use of marijuana, we contacted several organizations decidedly 'con' to medical marijuana — two of which were federal government agencies — and none knew of any voter initiatives or polls that were 'con' (50.01% or more con) to medical marijuana."

[106] Karen Tandy, "Marijuana: The Myths Are Killing Us," Police Chief Magazine, March 2005, available at [http://www.usdoj.gov/dea/pubs/pressrel/pr042605p.html].

[107] See, for example, J.G. Bachman et al., "Explaining Recent Increases in Students' Marijuana Use: Impacts of Perceived Risks and Disapproval, 1976 through 1996," American Journal of Public Health, vol. 88 (1998), pp. 887-892.

[108] Brief for the Drug Free America Foundation, Inc. et al. as Amici Curiae Supporting Petitioners at 26, Gonzales v. Raich, 125 S.Ct. 2195 (2005) (No. 03-1454).

[109] Ibid., at 27. The 1999 NHSDA was the first to include state-level estimates for various measures of drug use. Unfortunately, comprehensive state-level data prior to 1999 are not available from other sources.

[110] Care should be taken in comparing NHSDA data for 1999 with NSDUH data for 2002 and after, due to changes in survey methodology made in

2002. The trend observations drawn here from these data should therefore be considered suggestive rather than definitive.

[111] Dennis M. Gorman and J. Charles Huber, Jr., "Do Medical Cannabis Laws Encourage Cannabis Use?" *International Journal of Drug Policy*, vol. 18, no. 3 (May 2007), pp. 160- 167.

[112] Karen O'Keefe, et al., "Marijuana Use by Young People: The Impact of State Medical Marijuana Laws," updated June 2008, available at [http://www.mpp.org/teens]. (New Mexico was excluded from the study because it passed its law too recently.)

[113] U.S. General Accounting Office, Marijuana: Early Experiences with Four States' Laws That Allow Use for Medical Purposes, GAO-03-1 89, November 2002.

[114] Available at [http://www.usdoj .gov/dea/ongoing/calimarijuanap.html].

[115] U.S. General Accounting Office, Marijuana: Early Experiences with Four States' Laws That Allow Use for Medical Purposes, GAO-03-1 89, November 2002, p. 36.

[116] Ibid., p. 37.

[117] 117 Stuart Taylor, Jr., "Liberal Drug Warriors! Conservative Pot-Coddlers!," *National Journal*, June 11, 2005, p. 1738.

[118] Testimony of Thomas A. Constantine in U.S. Congress, Senate Committee on the Judiciary, Prescription for Addiction? The Arizona and California Medical Drug Use Initiatives, hearing, 104th Cong., 2nd sess., December 2, 1996 (Washington: GPO, 1997), pp. 42-43, 45.

[119] "Marijuana: Lawrence, Kansas, Ponders City Marijuana Ordinance — Impact of HEA Cited," available at [http://stopthedrugwar.org/chronicle/40 1/lawrence.shtml].

[120] Brief for U.S. Representative Mark E. Souder et al. as Amici Curiae Supporting Petitioners at 20, Gonzales v. Raich, 125 S.Ct. 2195 (2005) (No. 03-1454).

[121] "California Medical Marijuana Information," available on DEA's website at [http://www.usdoj .gov/dea/ongoing/calimarijuanap.html].

[122] U.S. General Accounting Office, Marijuana: Early Experiences with Four States' Laws That Allow Use for Medical Purposes, GAO-03-189, November 2002, p. 64. GAO interviewed 37 law enforcement agencies and found that the majority indicated that "medical-marijuana laws had not greatly affected their law enforcement activities." (p. 4)

[123] Eric Bailey, "CHP Revises Policy on Pot Seizures," Los Angeles Times (national edition), August 28, 2005, p. A12.

[124] Committee on Drugs and the Law, "Marijuana Should be Medically Available," Record of the Association of the Bar of the City of New York, vol. 52, no. 2 (March 1997), p. 238.

[125] Brief for the Leukemia and Lymphoma Society et al. as Amici Curiae Supporting Respondents at 1,2, Gonzales v. Raich, 125 S.Ct. 2195 (2005) (No. 03-1454).

[126] IOM Report, p. 18.

[127] 21 U.S.C. §844 and 18 U.S.C. §3571. 21 U.S.C. §844 also calls for a minimum fine of $1,000, and 21 U.S.C. §844a permits a civil penalty of up to $10,000.

[128] 21 U.S.C. §841(b)(1)(D).

[129] Communication from DEA Congressional Affairs to author dated September 27, 2005.

[130] Stacy Finz, "19 Named in Medicinal Pot Indictment, More than 9,300 Plants Were Seized in Raids," San Francisco Chronicle, June 24, 2005, p. B4.

[131] Lester Grinspoon and James B. Bakalar, "Marihuana as Medicine: A Plea for Reconsideration," *Journal of the American Medical Association*, vol. 273, no. 23 (June 21, 1995), p. 1876.

[132] Angel Wings Patient OutReach press release, November 29, 2004. Barnett represented Raich et al. in Supreme Court oral argument on this date.

[133] Brief for the States of California, Maryland, and Washington et al. as Amici Curiae Supporting Respondents at 3, Gonzales v. Raich, 125 S.Ct. 2195 (2005) (No. 03-1454).

[134] New State Ice Co. v. Liebmann, 285 U.S. 262, 311 (1932) (Brandeis, J., dissenting).

[135] Brief for the States of Alabama, Louisiana, and Mississippi et al. as Amici Curiae Supporting Respondents at 3, Gonzales v. Raich, 125 S.Ct. 2195 (2005) (No. 03-1454).

[136] Gonzales v. Raich, 125 S.Ct. 2195, 2220 (2005) (O'Connor, J., dissenting).

[137] Ibid. at 2229.

[138] Brief for the Drug Free America Foundation, Inc. et al. as Amici Curiae Supporting Petitioners at 12, Gonzales v. Raich, 125 S.Ct. 2195 (2005) (No. 03-1454).

[139] 21 U.S.C. §351-360

[140] Brief for Petitioners at 11, Gonzales v. Raich, 125 S.Ct. 2195 (2002) (No. 03-1454).

[141] Brief for Robert L. DuPont, M.D. et al. as Amici Curiae Supporting Petitioners at 19, Gonzales v. Raich, 125 S.Ct. 2195 (2005) (No. 03-1454).

[142] U.S. Food and Drug Administration, "Inter-Agency Advisory Regarding Claims That Smoked Marijuana Is a Medicine," press release, April 20, 2006, p. 1.

[143] See, for example, Lila Guterman, "The Dope on Medical Marijuana," Chronicle of Higher Education, June 2, 2000, p. A21.

[144] IOM Report, p. 14.

[145] "Federal Foolishness and Marijuana," *New England Journal of Medicine,* vol. 336, no. 5 (January 30, 1997), p. 366.

[146] Chuck Thomas, Marijuana Policy Project press release dated April 20, 1999, available at [http://www.mpp.org/releases/nr042099.html].

[147] Brief for the Drug Free America Foundation, Inc. et al. as Amici Curiae Supporting Petitioners at 9, Gonzales v. Raich, 125 S.Ct. 2195 (2005) (No. 03-1454).

[148] For example, the amici curiae brief of the Drug Free America Foundation et al. reveals this history to discredit the medical marijuana movement (pp. 9-11). Actually, NORML and some other drug reform organizations are open in acknowledging that they support patient access to marijuana as a first step toward decriminalizing or legalizing marijuana for use by adults in general. See, for example, Joab Jackson, "Medical Marijuana: From the Fringe to the Forefront," Baltimore City Paper, March 28, 2002, [http://www.alternet.org/drugreporter/127 14].

[149] Barry R. McCaffrey, "We're on a Perilous Path," Newsweek, February 3, 1997, p. 27.

[150] Lester Grinspoon and James B. Bakalar, "Marihuana as Medicine: A Plea for Reconsideration," *Journal of the American Medical Association,* vol. 273, no. 23 (June 21, 1995), p. 1876.

[151] Quoted in MSNBC.com story, "Western States Back Medical Marijuana," November 4, 2004, available at [http://msnbc.msn.com/id/6406453].

INDEX

U

T

V

W